# The Caregiver Resource Manual

## By

## Julie V. Kallal

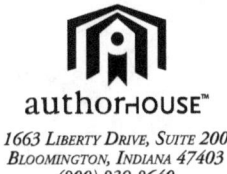

authorHOUSE™

1663 LIBERTY DRIVE, SUITE 200
BLOOMINGTON, INDIANA 47403
(800) 839-8640
WWW.AUTHORHOUSE.COM

First published by AuthorHouse 7/25/2006

ISBN: 1-4208-6292-8 (sc)

Printed in the United States of America
Bloomington, Indiana

This book is printed on acid-free paper.

# Acknowledgement

## A Special Thank You Note

**A** *well thought appreciation and gratitude message to those whose lives I touch!*

**S**aying *a sincere and meaningful thank you and appreciation to many dedicated*
**P**eople *who share my honest commitment and devotion is not an easy task. The*
**E**nhancement *and provision of service in caring for those with special needs,*
**C**hildren *and the elderly in our modern society is a great undertaking. In the*
**I**nterest *of compassion and love, this manual is a distillation of the cooperative*
**A**ctions *of many individuals – colleagues, teachers, learners, consultants and*
**L**oving *members of my family. To them, I dedicate this noble Manual of Care.*

**T**o *Anthony, my husband, Nick and Tony, my children, Nellie, my sister, Chiara*
**H**azel *and Charmaine, my nieces, Nap, Danny and Mike, my brothers, my staff,*
**A**nnette, *Theya, Deo, Judith, Jeancy, Bernadette, Gigi, Jigs, my TTMC class,*
**N**amely *Raquel, Edwin, Lennie, Andy, Ma. Christina, Mars, Celina, Felicisima,*
**K**laire *with a C, Gelvin, Elmer, Gloria and Er... a big bouquet of love and thanks!*

**Y**earning *to make a difference in how to facilitate a course, hoping to impart*
**O**utstanding *and state of the art methods and techniques in caring for children,*
**U**nderstanding *the wishes of those with special needs are enclosed in the book.*

**N**ow *for my special message to my select readers, the would be caregivers all*
**O**ver *the world – We provide the answer to satisfy you for a while, then we*
**T**each *the process to satisfy you for life! Remember, the strength and beauty*
**E**volve *from our unity and unique diversity. May the Lord bless us always!*

***Julie V. Kallal, B.Sc, B.Ed., M.Ed.***
*Worldwide Caregiving Consultant*
*CEO and Dean of Further Education*
*SICES International*

Jacquelyn Paterno
Layout and Format

Robert Streatch
Digital Illustrations

Donna Marchyshyn
Artwork and Illustrations

## SICES Mission and Vision

We believe that children are our future
Teach them well and let them lead the way
Show them all the beauty they possess inside
Give them a sense of pride
To make it easier, let the children's laughter
Remind us how we used to be

We believe that seniors shape our future
Care for them and let them guide the way
Let them share the beauty they possess inside
Give them a sense of pride
To make it easier, let the senior's laughter
Remind them how they used to be

Disabled decided long ago
Never to walk in anyone's shadow
If they fail, if they succeed
At least they live as they believe
No matter what we take from them
We can't take away their dignity

Because the greatest care of all
Is happening to us
We've found the greatest
Care of all inside of us.

The greatest care of all
Is easy to achieve
Learning to give our care
Is the greatest care of all
So if by chance that special place
    [ C A N A D A?]
That we've been dreaming of
Leads us to happiness
THEN WE'VE ACHIEVED
OUR NOBLE GOAL
THE GREATEST LOVE AND CARE OF ALL

*Music: The Greatest Love of All*
*Lyrics modified by: Julie V. Kallal*

## Declaration of Care

We are the children of the world
We know nothing but laughter and play
We sing, we smile, we cry but we try
To learn the teaching that you give
So we rely on the care that you bring

We are the aged of the world
We know nothing but dream of the pleasures
When life gave us the essence of youth
We ache, we hurt, we cry, we rebel
So we rely on the care that you bring

We are the crippled of the world
We know nothing but fear and pain
We stare but we cannot talk
We listen but we cannot hear
We walk only to fall again and again
So we rely on the care that you bring

We are the caregivers of the world
We bring laughter and happiness and hope
Today is the time to be carefree
No matter how young, how crippled, and how old
Today, we bring to those we care,
all the blessings and teachings and skills
SICES International has given us to share!

*Julie V. Kallal*

# MAIN TABLE OF CONTENTS

# TABLE OF MODULES

# HOW TO'S

# *The Training Standards*

## 1. THE LIVE-IN CAREGIVER PROGRAM

The Program is designed to bring workers to Canada who will provide child care, elderly care or care of the disabled, without supervision, in a private home on a temporary basis. The program called "The live-in Caregiver Program" also known as the "LCP" has replaced the Foreign Domestic Movement program on April 27, 1992.

## 2. THE LIVE-IN CAREGIVER REQUIREMENTS

A LIVE-IN CAREGIVER MEANS A PERSON WHO WILL BE HIRED TO PROVIDE CHILD CARE, SENIOR HOME SUPPORT CARE OR CARE OF THE DISABLED, WITHOUT SUPERVISION, IN A PRIVATE HOUSEHOLD. A LIVE-IN CAREGIVER IS REQUIRED TO LIVE IN THE EMPLOYER'S HOME.

**EDUCATION** – the live-in caregiver must complete a course of study that is equivalent to a successful completion of a Canadian secondary school or 12 years of formal education

**TRAINING OR EXPERIENCE** – applicants must have either training or work experience in a field or occupation related to the employment in Canada.

* TRAINING: successful completion of six months of full-time training in a **classroom setting**. OR

* EXPERIENCE: one year of full-time paid employment, including at least six months of continuous employment with one employer, within the last three years of the date of application.

Care of family members, volunteer work experience, or personal experience as a parent is not considered eligible employment.

Employment must be related to the job offer in Canada. For example, if the job in Canada is to care for a person with a disability, the caregiver applicant's knowledge and skills must be related to this type of care.

**LANGUAGE** – the ability to speak, read and understand English or French at a level sufficient to communicate effectively in an unsupervised setting.

**MEDICAL AND SECURITY** – the Canadian health and security requirements.

3. **INSTRUCTOR'S QUALIFICATION:**

⇒ Must be a graduate of any degree specializing in behavioral science, paramedical field, social sciences or education.

⇒ Must have practised his specific field for at least a year.

⇒ Must have at least a year of teaching experience.

⇒ Must possess a pleasant disposition and patience and exhibit effective communication.

⇒ Must have undergone the SICES Six Month Live-in Caregiver Course/

⇒ Must have undergone the Instructor's Seminar given by the Program Director.

4. **TRAINEE'S QUALIFICATIONS:**

⇒ Must be between 18 to 55 years of age.

⇒ Must have finished (successfully completed) at least 12 years of formal education.

⇒ Must have a working knowledge of the English language.

⇒ Must submit the following:

    ⇒ 4 pieces of 2" x 2" photo

    ⇒ Payments of Tuition Fee

    ⇒ Police Clearance

    ⇒ Academic Records

5. **THE LIVE-IN CAREGIVER PROGRAM**

**Q1:** There is a shortage of caregivers in Canada.

**A1:** False. There is no shortage of caregivers in Canada. Generally however, there is a shortage of **LIVE-IN** caregivers in Canada.

**Q2:** The Live-in Caregiver Program is designed to bring workers to Canada on a temporary basis for certain kinds of live-in employment.

**A2:** True. Care of the child, care of the elderly or care of the disabled. Care of the home is no longer included as a job requiring out of country help.

**Q3:** What is the difference between VISITOR'S VISA (TOURIST VISA) and EMPLOYMENT VISA (EMPLOYMENT AUTHORIZATION)?

**A3:**   There are two visas in order to work or study in Canada. You must be eligible first to come as a visitor meaning that you can travel in Canada. The second visa is your status meaning length of stay and work permit and study permit. Under the new ruling, visitors to Canada can take non-credit courses under six months without requiring a study visa.

PLEASE NOTE THAT UNDER THE NEW RULING, COURSES THAT TAKE 6 MONTHS OR UNDER NO LONGER REQUIRE STUDENT AUTHORIZATION JUST A VISITOR VISA.

**Q4:**   What are the three main requirements to qualify under the LCP?
**A4:**   1. successful completion of the equivalent of a Canadian High School education
    **OR**
   2. six months full time caregiving training **OR** twelve months of experience in a paid employment in an **occupation** related to the job that is being offered within the last 3 years of application.
   3. ability to speak, read and understand either the English or French language.

**Q5:**   Since a college degree has more years than a Canadian high school diploma, there is no need for a college graduate to undergo the six month training as a live-in caregiver.
**A5:**   False. If an individual has a degree with a program that does not meet the job requirements for live-in caregivers (i.e. child care, geriatric care or care of the disabled), then the individual must undergo training or must have proof of experience in the job that is being sought.

**Q6:**   A domestic helper who has worked in Hong Kong for the past 5 years as a housekeeper will have no problems in satisfying the training or experience requirements of the LCP.
**A6:**   False. The applicant will fail since she has **no experience within the last three years** in care of the child, the elderly or the disabled. Under the LCP program, housekeeping is no longer a major consideration. The prospective employer must either require a caregiver for the child, the elderly or the disabled. Even if she had some caregiving experience but the experience was beyond three years from the date of application, she would not qualify.

**Q7:**   Caregivers hired under the LCP can provide child care, senior care or care of the disabled anywhere in Canada.'
**A7:**   False. The key word is **live-in** and the employment authorization spells out the **specific employer and location.**

**Q8:** An employment authorization is usually valid for one year.

**A8:** True. The employment authorization is issued by Immigration Canada allowing the caregiver to work or change employers while in Canada. Permission must be obtained when changing employers. Remember that a valid work authorization must be in the caregiver's possession before starting another live-in employment. Trial employment is illegal.

**Q9:** Both the caregiver and the employer must be aware that the caregiver is free to change employer and the employer is free to change employee at anytime during the employment authorization period with valid reasons.

**A9:** True.

**Q10:** Employment and Immigration Canada can intervene on the caregiver's behalf if there was an employer-employee dispute.

**A10:** False. Employment and Immigration Canada is not a party to an employment contract, therefore it has no authority to intervene in the employer-employee relationship or to enforce the terms and conditions of employment. The Provincial Labour Standards however can interfere with regards to the terms and conditions of employment.

**Q11:** If a caregiver lost her offer of employment while training, where can she go for employment assistance?

**A11:** - friends and/or relatives who are now in Canada or
- depend on classmates with offers of employment (to act as possible source of employer contracts)
- SICES Canada (only for SICES trainees or graduates whose offer either expired or terminated) . Remember that SICES Philippines is strictly a training center and it is illegal for it to act as a recruitment or employment center. SICES Canada, on the other hand, is in the business of training and referral services.

**Q12:** Please outline the procedure once a prospective employer applies for a caregiver.

**A12:** 1. The employer fills out an APPLICATION FOR A LIVE-IN CAREGIVER obtainable at the nearest Human Resource Development Centre (HRDC). A copy should be retained by the employer.
2. Once completed, the form should be submitted back to the HRDC. The submitted form should contain proof that there are no local caregivers available. A copy of a major newspaper ad should accompany the application form.
3. Sometimes, HRDC may recommend unemployed caregivers who are already in Canada.

4. Processing may take 30 to 90 days for out of country application because HRDC gives priority processing for caregivers who are already in Canada.

5. If the application is approved, the employer receives a CONFIRMED OFFER OF EMPLOYMENT from Immigration Canada in Vegreville, Alberta via HRDC.

6. A copy of the Authenticated or Confirmed Offer is sent to its post abroad.

7. The post abroad, depending on how busy the office is, notifies the applicant by sending an APPLICATION KIT together with a letter informing the applicant of an Offer of Employment.

8. Once the application form is received by the applicant, he or she has 90 days to comply with the requirements.

9. Once the completed application is received back by the Canadian post, an interviews is scheduled.

10. If the interview is successful, a Visitor's Visa with an Employment Authorization is issued.

11. Depending on how busy the Canadian post abroad is and how complete your submitted documents are, the entire process may take from 2 months to a year.

**Q13.** Once in Canada under the Live-in Caregiver Program, what are some of the rights of the caregiver?

**A13:**  a. The caregiver cannot work for any other employer other than the person stipulated on the contract.

    b. The caregiver must live-in but can from time to time (e.g. days off or some evenings) spend the night with friends or relatives.

    c. The caregiver can look for another caregiving job (permission must be obtained from Immigration Canada to work for another employer) if irrevocable differences occur affecting employment. The employer can also terminate the caregiver's employment with good reasons.

    d. The caregiver can apply for unemployment benefit (approx. 75% of salary) if no jobs are available.
(Note that the caregiver contributes towards her Income Tax, Canada Pension and Employment Insurance every month. Similarly, the employer contributes towards Canada Pension and 1.4 % towards Employment Insurance).

    e. The caregiver, after two years of continuous employment, can apply for a landed immigrant status and can apply for his or her family to come to Canada as permanent residents or immigrants.

    f. While waiting for the immigrant status to be approved, the caregiver may be issued an "Open Visa" meaning that he or she can now work for any other employment open to residents of Canada.

**Q14:** What if a member of the family is disqualified under the Immigration Act.

**A14:** The principal applicant (the caregiver) almost always applies to become a permanent resident. The members of her immediate family i.e., spouse, children (legitimate or not – so long as they have been identified in the Family Composition Form which was filled out during the initial Caregiver Application outside of Canada) will be included in the application for permanent residency. However, certain criteria must again be adhered to. The most critical are the medical and criminal check requirements. If the caregiver or any of the sponsored members do not meet the criteria, the caregiver's application for immigrant status is denied and the caregiver must leave Canada.

**Q15:** What are two major disqualification criteria for the caregiver's family members?

**A15:** **Medical Condition** that will place a strain on the Health Program of Canada (e.g. Aids, Cancer. Note that Tuberculosis is considered curable and is not considered an inadmissible disease. It must be cured completely however, before the application is considered)
**Criminals such as** – murderers, drug addicts, rapists, armed robbers, sex molesters.

**Q16:** Can I, during my authorized employment, return to my country for a vacation?

**A16:** Yes, get a letter from your employer permitting you to go. The letter should specify the duration and the employer's commitment to have you back as an employee. Such a letter will expedite the issuing of a re-entry visa. Note what is stamped in your VISA (Multiple – you can exit and come back; Single Entry – you must obtain another entry to Canada). If you remain outside Canada at or after the expiration of your employment authorization, you will have to re-apply to Canada under the Live-in Caregiver Program.

**Q17:** The live-in caregiver has the same legal rights as Canadians in terms of working condition and fair treatment from employers.

**A17:** True.

**Q18:** Employment Standards regulations may cover rights in areas such as:
a. vacation time with pay    c. maximum charges for room and board
b. overtime pay                  d. minimum wage         e. paid public holidays

**A18:** True.

**Q19:** Employment Standards can change the terms and conditions stipulated in the employment authorization.

**A19:** False. Labor and Employment Standards can only help in enforcing the employment contract but cannot change the terms and conditions stipulated in the contract.

**Q20:** "Time off is not yours to spend as you wish." The employer can demand the caregiver to give up her time off.

**A20:** False. Live-in caregivers have the same legal rights as Canadians in terms of fair working conditions and fair treatment from their employers.

**Q21:** While working, an employer contributes the appropriate portion of his own money outside of the caregiver's pay towards Employment Insurance and Canada Pension Premium.

**A21:** True.

**Q22:** If the caregiver loses his job for no fault on his part, he will be asked to leave Canada.

**A22:** False. Since an employment authorization, issued by Immigration Canada (not the employer) is valid for one year, Immigration Canada will allow an unemployed caregiver to look for another job or even apply for unemployment benefits in the event there are no jobs available. The caregiver should ensure that his VISA has not expired though.

**Q23:** The caregiver should always ask for a Record of Employment (ROE) from her employer whenever she quits her job.

**A23:** True. A Record of Employment is a proof of employment and is required if a caregiver wishes to draw unemployment benefits. It is also required by Immigration Canada when the caregiver applies for immigrant status after two years of continuous contract. The caregiver may have a hard time tracking down employers who move so it is recommended to get an ROE upon termination . A caregiver can also request the ROE office to help obtain a record of employment from the employer.

**Q24:** A live-in caregiver needs at least 2 years of continuous employment before he or she can apply for a permanent residence in Canada.

**A24:** True

**Q25:** Please clarify the meaning of continuous employment.

**A25:** 1. Continuous employment does not mean employment from one employer only for two years.

The Immigration Act allows a caregiver to complete two years of employment in three years of stay under the Live-in Caregiver Program to qualify for a permanent residence status.

If the caregiver for example, loses his job and was not able to work again until two months later, then those two months must be made up at the end of two years, in other words, his application will be considered after 26 months rather than 24 months.

**Q26:** What happens if the caregiver cannot fulfill 24 months of work in three years time.

**A26:** The application for permanent residence may be denied and the caregiver must leave the country and re-apply as a caregiver again. The count down for 24 months of employment starts all over.

**Q27:** Once a caregiver receives a favourable assessment on his permanent residence application, he may apply for an open employment authorization (popularly known as an Open Visa) and may take any job available for Canadians.

**A27:** True.

**Q28:** Once a permanent residence status is obtained, the caregiver can begin to assist non-immediate family members from abroad to apply to come to Canada.

**A28:** True.

**Q29:** Once the caregiver gains two years of employment as a live-in caregiver, she can automatically sponsor her family as permanent residents.

**A29:** True. The caregiver's application for permanent residence includes her immediate family (criteria specifics)

**Q30:** How many hours is considered average per month?

**A30:** The minimum wage is based on an average of 205 hours per month or 9.5 per day.

**Q31:** Can the caregiver who has applied for an immigrant status be denied.

**A31:** Yes, he has to satisfy Canada Immigration that he can be an asset as a citizen of Canada through proofs of, among others:
- ⇒ legal employment
- ⇒ no police record
- ⇒ enough savings
- ⇒ eligibility of sponsored members
- ⇒ volunteer activities

**Q32:** What happens if the caregiver or a member of her sponsored family does not qualify under permanent status.

**A32:** The caregiver will be asked to leave Canada.

**Q33:** A caregiver applying for a job in Canada can be denied because of:

**A33:** a. over qualifications   a: False. The more qualified you are the better chances of passing.

b. he or she is married with or without children.  b. False

c. he or she is single with children.  c. False

d. he or she is related to the prospective employer. d. False. Although the program has been abused by those who bring in their relatives for convenience, legitimate employers should not have any difficulty in satisfying the HRDC requirements.

e. she or he did not comply with the three requirements (education, training or experience, English fluency) e. True

f: no compliance with the training requirement.  f: True (length and quality of caregiving training must be at least 750 hours, 5 days/ week, 6 months or 26 weeks, in classroom setting, accredited by local government)

**Q34:** Is there a minimum wage recommendation for caregivers.

**A34:** Yes, each province has it's own minimum wage for caregivers. See Sample for Alberta on Q: 37

**Q35:** How is vacation pay calculated?

**A35:** *4% of regular wages for lesser period than 12 months.
*Two weeks pay after 12 months of employment

**Q36:** As a tourist, can I enroll in the Six Month LCP course while in Canada.

**A36:** Under the new immigration ruling, tourists can now take the 6 month course without obtaining a student authorizations. Short courses 6 months and under no longer require student authorization. However, you must make arrangement with the school so that upon entry, you can start the course if it's 6 months. You will not be permitted to take a six month course if you have already been in Canada for a while. You will then need to obtain a student visa and must leave Canada to obtain it.

**Q37:** Can the caregiver after 12 months of work leave Canada for a holiday and come back again?

**A37:** No, the letter of employment is for one year only. The caregiver must always have a valid visitor's visa to leave Canada, otherwise, he or she must apply again. The employment authorization is renewable every year so before the expiry date (one year to date of employment), the employer must re-apply Canada Immigration.

**Q38:** Please give a detailed calculation of how a salary is paid and the deductions required including employer's contribution. I understand that different provinces have different rates.

**A38:** Using the 2001 Salary for Caregivers in Alberta:

## REVENUE CANADA INFORMATION

Each province has its own guidelines for wages. Contact the nearest HRDC (Human Resource Development Center for each province)

### Sample of Live –in Caregiver's Wages (Alberta, 2004)

CHILDREN

| Sample Wages of Live-in Caregiver for Children (Alberta, 2004) | | | | | |
|---|---|---|---|---|---|
| | Employee's Contribution | Employer's Contribution | Due to Receiver General | Gross Wage | Net Wage |
| Gross Wage | | | | 1405.84 | |
| | | | | | |
| Particulars | | | | | |
| Canada Pension Plan (CPP) | 55.15 | 55.15 | 110.3 | | |
| Employment Insurance | 27.84 | 38.98 | 66.82 | | |
| Tax | | | 119.15 | | |
| Federal | 106.05 | | | | |
| Provincial | 13.1 | | | | |
| Room & Board | 300 | | | | |
| Total | 502.14 | 94.13 | 296.27 | | 903.7 |

| Sample Wages of Live-in Caregiver for the Elderly or Persons with Special Needs (Alberta, 2004) | | | | | |
|---|---|---|---|---|---|
| | Employee's Contribution | Employer's Contribution | Due to Receiver General | Gross Wage | Net Wage |
| Gross Wage | | | | $1646.67 | |
| | | | | | |
| Particulars | | | | | |
| Canada Pension Plan (CPP) | $88.23 | $80.23 | $160.46 | | |
| Employment Insurance | $37.87 | $53.02 | $90.89 | | |
| Tax | | | $240.65 | | |
| Federal | $181.10 | | | | |
| Provincial | $59.55 | | | | |
| Room & Board | $300.00 | | | | |
| Total | $666.75 | $133.25 | $492.00 | | $979.92 |

*Note:*

The live-in caregiver may be paid semi-monthly (15th and end of the month) or monthly (end of the month)

Remittance to Revenue Canada must be paid on or before the 15th of the month following the month of pay.

Employer bookkeeping is simple – 24 entries per year (payroll & revenue Canada).

T4 summary report and slip/s are to be filed before the end of February

## 6. THE CAREGIVER PROGRAM GOAL:

To prepare course participants in obtaining a caregiver certificate that meets Canada Immigration criteria for its Live-in Caregiver Program and to equip participants with the required competencies for CAREGIVING as a career.

## 7. COURSE DESCRIPTION:
The LCP course was specifically designed and developed for the trainees to be equipped with the working **knowledge,** relevant and essential **skills** and the proper **attitudes (KSA)** required by the job.

**COURSE CURRICULUM:** The course was specifically designed and developed based on a competency based curriculum that complies strictly on SICES COMPETENCY STANDARDS. In short the curriculum ensures that the graduates are competent, i.e. the workers are equipped not only with the working **KNOWLEDGE,** and relevant and essential **SKILLS** but also with the proper and professional **ATTITUDES (KSA)** required for the job.

**COURSE DURATION:** Six months (four weeks a month at five days a week) 750 hours classroom setting. Some training centers will add a practicuum (field practice) to the course but this field practice to hone the in classroom skills in caregiving is not considered in the determining the length of the course as a compliance to the 750 hour requirements of Canada Immigration.

**THE COMPETENCY BASED COURSE (Knowledge, Skills and Attitudes)**

The course in addressing the above **KSA** comes in six modules as follows:

MODULE 1  The Training Induction, Personality Enhancement, Effective Communication and Coping Mechanism

      Module 1 is a 120 hour course completed in a month

and deals with the training induction, course expectation, personality enhancement, cultural adaptation and effective communication.

MODULE 2    Health and Safety, First Aid and CPR, Medication Administration and Proper Food Handling and Storage

Module 2 is a 120 hour course completed in a month and deals with Health and Safety issues such as prevention, illnesses and diseases of children, adults and persons with special needs, and medicine administration. The module also leads to a First Aid and CPR certificate.

MODULE 3    Home Management, Nutrition, Proper Basic Food Preparation and the Art of Meal Presentation

Module 3 is a 120 hour course completed in a month and deals with concept of home time management using effective use of schedules of house chores, basic nutrition and meal preparation. Basic to this module is an understanding that this is a secondary to personal and nursing care, skills training.

MODULE 4    Care for the Child

Module 4 is a 120 hour course completed in a month and deals with the philosophy of child care, the various roles of a caregiver and provision for the needs and activities of children including procedure for reporting child abuse.

MODULE 5    Care for the Elderly and Person with Special Needs

Module 5 is a 120 hour course completed in a month and deals with the rights of the elderly and the disabled (person with special needs), the needs and activities of the elderly and disabled, the various roles of the caregivers and hands-on skills on personal and basic nursing care of the elderly and disabled.

MODULE 6    Future Employment in Canada

Module 6 is a 120 hour course completed in a month and deals with their future employer; a thorough understanding of the community. The participant will be living in; an understanding of the Rights and Freedom of the Caregiver while at work and on days off, and the personal profile of the specific person requiring care in terms of the requirements of needs and activities.

**WRAP UP WEEK**

Review of Module Objectives

Questions and Answers on Modules

Written Evaluation on

The Module

The Materials

The Instructors

Recommendations

Day 1 – Modules 1 & 2 Q & A, Review of Objectives, Evaluation

Day 2 – Module 3 & 4 ditto

Day 3 – Module 5 & 6 ditto

Day 4 – Oral interaction / Mock Interview

Day 5 – Completion and Submission of Requirements

## 8. HOME SETTING PRACTICE:

It is a 120 hour course completed in 3 weeks and deals with the practice of personal care of the caregiver to a child, elderly and person with special needs in selected private homes.

## 9. COMPONENTS OF THE COURSE

The 750 hour course is composed of two components: (See also course outline)

* The Theoretical Studies Component – aimed at providing the theoretical knowledge, theories and notes on caregiving in general.

* The Skills Training Component – provides the trainees the opportunity to learn and experience the various skills and working knowledge vital in performing the job of the caregiver. It is an in-center activity and focuses on the honing of critical skills in the following modules:

⇒ Personality Enhancement, Effective Communication and Cultural Adaptation

⇒ Health and Safety, First-Aid & CPR

⇒ Home Management, Nutrition, Canada Food Guide, Basic Food Preparation and Meal Presentation

⇒ Care of the Child

⇒ Care of the Elderly/Disabled

⇒ Preparation for Future Employment

## 10. GOALS AND OBJECTIVES OF THE COURSE

The overall goal of the course is to obtain the appropriate certification in order to gain initial employment in Canada.

### COURSE OBJECTIVES
Upon completion of the course, the participants must be able to:

- observe and demonstrate safe and desirable work habits, attitudes and behaviour;
- describe the role of a caregiver in relation to a child, an elderly and disabled;
- describe the social, physical, intellectual, creative, cultural, and emotional needs, development, and activities of infants, pre-schoolers and school aged children;
- describe the social, physical, intellectual, creative, cultural, economic and emotional needs and activities of the elderly and the disabled;
- attend to the needs and activities of the individuals described above;
- operate equipment and tools relevant to the job as a caregiver;
- perform household chores using daily, weekly and monthly schedules;
- perform first aid and/or CPR and describe proper procedure of alerting the medical system;
- prepare foods appropriate for the child, the elderly or the disabled;
- prepare and administer medications as prescribed for the child, the elderly or the disabled;
- perform activities necessary for the health and safety of the child, the elderly or the disabled;
- describe the required and appropriate materials and consumable used by a caregiver.

## 11. COURSE METHODOLOGY:
The method that is employed is to assure that participants achieve the Live-in Caregiver Course professional responsibility. The method selected can range from instructor directed to student managed to directed.

**The Instructor Directed Method** - the instructor controls the program. The instructor make the decision regarding how content and skills are to be acquired. The instructor's energy.

**The Student Managed Method**, the learners make a number of decisions about the application of edge and skills within the guidelines established by the instructor. The learners have definite responsibilities. The instructor becomes the facilitator and an information giver.

**The Student Directed Method** is at the other end of the continuum from the instructor directed method. Instructor plays the role of facilitator and learners are responsible for their learning. This method requires that students are capable of managing their own time, are self-motivated and have had previous exposure to and experiencing learning.

An effective combination of teaching methods is recommended and a variety of teaching/learning strategies be employed. Learners should be provided with the opportunity to develop decision-making and problem skills and become lifelong learners. Incorporating learner responsibilities into the live-in caregiver course is this goal.

Those teaching/learning strategies which: allow for the greatest active participation of the learners, provide the greatest degree of reality or accuracy (experiential), and are of personal interest to the learners.

## 12.  TEACHING/LEARNING STRATEGIES

### DEMONSTRATIONS

This strategy can be used by instructors and learners. They can be very helpful in promoting optimum learning situations. They can be used to show procedures (how to vacuum, scramble eggs, set tables, bathe an infant), to explain new techniques (first aid & CPR) or to incorporate laboratory lessons that would be too expensive for a large group of students to complete individually (roast beef, turkey). However, it is frequently better not to give a demonstration than to give one that is poorly executed.

The following outlines a list of teaching/learning strategies that are recommended. You are encouraged to utilize internal teaching/learning strategies that support and promote the achievement of the goals and objectives of the Caregiver Course Curriculum.

1.  Class discussions (instructor/learner)
2.  Activity sheets
3.  Field trips
4.  Independent Study
5.  Brainstorming
6.  Mind mapping
7.  Case Studies
8.  Syndicated work films, filmstrip, videos
9.  Field trips
10. Collages, scrapbooks
14. Displays
15. Games
16. Role playing
17. Group projects
18. Small group
19. Community project
20. Bulletin board/porters
21. Resource personnel
22. Student research, essays
23. Instructor checklists

11. Panel discussions
12. Debate/interviews
13. Creative writing

24. Individual presentation
25, Anecdotes, observations
26. Demonstration

## 13.  EVALUATION AND ASSESSMENT

Evaluation appraises the nature and worth of something. Evaluation applies to what is taught (the program) while assessment applies to what is learned (the learner's experience). However, in this manual evaluation applies equally to what is taught (the program) and what is learned (the learner's experience. Learner's growth must be evaluated in each module in order to measure the degree to which learner has met the objectives. Instructors need to find out what the learners are learning, and the learners must be informed of their progress. Arrangement for learner evaluation should be a part of program planning.

In planning for learner evaluation, the instructor must assess individual scores to correspond with class time planned. For example, if a major project is expected to take one half of the module time to complete, the score for that project should comprise one half of the module's final mark.

Evaluation instruments should be **valid, reliable and usable** for the nature of the learning activity. Learners should know how this work and effort will be assessed as they begin each module.

Accurate records of learner achievement marks must be maintained and recorded.

## CHARACTERISTICS OF GOOD EVALUATION

Evaluation facilities self-evaluation. The learner develops a healthy self-concept, acceptance and respect of his uniqueness and that of others.

Evaluation is an integral part of the teaching/learning process. For example, a discussion of eating patterns may appraise a learner's awareness of nutrition. This appraisal may be used in the planning of future lessons.

Evaluation is concerned with processes as well as outcomes. The means should justify the end. Evaluation is a continuing process not simply a test result.

## LEVELS OF EVALUATION
The course employs three levels of evaluation as follows:

— **Reaction Level Evaluation** is undertaken through administering a prepared evaluation instrument to elicit from the participants areas in which the course needs to enhance in terms of its administration and management, the course contents and objectives, the training materials provided.

— **Learning Level Evaluation** is done through the use of achievement test (both practical and written), teacher observations, peer group evaluations and administered to the trainees during the conduct and at the end of the course.

— **Performance Level Evaluation** is done through skills tests or the competency based test.

## PLANNING FOR EVALUATION

A useful approach is to identify valid evaluation procedures for each objective in a module.

The first step would be to prepare a course grid which indicates:
1. the modules in a course
2. the time allotment for each module.

The use of a grid should help the instructor:
1. in keeping a clear perspective on what is happening or should be happening in a module.
2. in evaluating, decision making, problem solving or analyzing activities.

## OBJECTIVES OF ASSESSMENT

1. To assess the degree to which the learner has met the objectives
2. To assess individual learner needs, thereby providing the basis for continuation, remediation, enrichment (Example: oral quizzing, First Aid Make up test)
3. To use the results of the assessment as a basis for feedback to the learner on his progress or instructor on follow-ups.
4. To provide meaningful data for reporting individual learner's progress (e.g. employer)
5. To provide guidelines and information for student self-motivation, direction and professional growth.
6. To determine learner's course entry and exit behaviors.
7. To measure knowledge and skills gained in the three domains of learning:

- AFFECTIVE - personal growth and attitudes
- COGNITIVE - knowledge and understanding of concepts
- PSYCHOMOTOR- products and manipulation skills

## EVALUATION/ASSESSMENT TECHNIQUES AND SAMPLES

### 1. COGNITIVE (THEORY & KNOWLEDGE)

Test can be:
- oral (instructor/learner interaction)
- practical (food presentation)
- written
  - multiple choice
  - true or false
  - matching type
  - sentence completion
  - cloze tests
  - short answers
  - essays
  - research

### 2. AFFECTIVE (PERSONAL GROWTH)

In this area, it is difficult to be objective. However, evaluation in the affective domain should be continuous and ongoing. Some means to identify and appraise behaviors by both instructors and learners are:

- attitude questionnaires questions
- journals or course diary questions
- anecdotal reporting
- forced choice
- open ended
- interviewing

### 3. PSYCHOMOTOR (MANIPULATIVE SKILL/END PRODUCT)

- Specific skills should be identified. Products or exercises must be chosen which will utilize these skills. Evaluation should be in terms of the extent to which students develop these identified skills.

- With any product/skill evaluation, expected standards must identified
- before work begins/ components of skill evaluation may include:

  ■ learner's work habits in relation to the equipment and materials

  ■ cooperation with others

  ■ use of resources(human or facilities)

- time required for completion

- accuracy

- final product/performance

## THE LIVE-IN CAREGIVER COURSE
## COURSE OUTLINE

| MODULE TITLE | HOURS |
|---|---|
| • Training Induction (Training Standards)<br>• Personality Enhancement<br>• Effective Communication<br>• Work Values/Coping Mechanisms | 120 |
| • Home and Personal Health and Safety<br>• First Aid & CPR (Cardio-Pulmonary Resuscitation)<br>• Medicine Administration<br>• Proper Food Handling and Storage | 120 |
| • Home Management (Theory and Class Laboratory)<br>• Nutrition (Nutrients and Their Functions)<br>• Basic Food/Meal Preparation<br>• Various Food/Meal Presentation | 120 |
| • Care for the Child (Theory and Critical Skills Development) | 120 |
| • Care of the Elderly and Person with Special Needs (Theory and Critical Skills Development) | 120 |
| • SPECIAL PROJECT: MY FUTURE EMPLOYMENT<br>• Cultural Adaptation (The Acculturation Process) | 120 |
| **WRAP UP WEEK** | 30 |
| **TOTAL** | 750 |

## HOW THE COURSE IS CONDUCTED
1. A new module is scheduled each month as follows:
   **Week 1& 2 :** Course Objectives, Theoretical Studies (Knowledge), Modeling of Critical Skills, Instructor's Demonstrations, Individual and Group

Assignments of Presentations and Projects and Film Viewing.

**Week 3:** Individual Task Practice of Critical Skills,   Individual and Group Work and Class presentations.

**Week 4:** One-on- one assessment /Group Test/Make up/ Submission of Assignments

2.  A new student may register anytime but may not start until the beginning of next month.  Example: A trainee may start with Module 5 and end with Module 4.
3.  Attendance is compulsory and all lessons are in classroom settings.
4.  Initial one-on-one assessment of critical skills are included in the tuition fee however, repeats (passing mark is 80%)  cost extra to defray the cost of materials and instructor's time.

## WRAP UP WEEK

>Review of Module Objectives  > Questions and Answers on Modules
>Written Evaluation on  * The Module *The Materials * The instructors *
Recommendations
Day 1 - Module 1 & 2 Q & A, Review of Objectives, Evaluation
Day 2 - Module 3 & 4 Q & A, Review of Objectives, Evaluation
Day 3 - Module 5 & 6  Q&A, Review of Objectives, Evaluation
Day 4 - Picture taking, clearance, issuance of certificates
Day 5 – Graduation and Socialization

# MODULE 1
## PERSONALITY ENHANCEMENT, CULTURAL ADAPTATION
## AND EFFECTIVE COMMUNICATION MODULE
## TIME ALLOTED - 120 HOURS

TERMINAL OBJECTIVES OF MODULE 1

Upon completion of Module 1, the participant will be able to:
- explain personality
- identify positive and negative personality traits
- create his own SPICE profile using assessment of self as well as feedback from significant others
- explain the acculturation process
- appreciate the impact of acculturation
- appreciate the HOST COUNTRY AND ITS PEOPLE
- appreciate CANADA, ITS GEOGRAPHY, FACTS AND FIGURES
- practise effective communication
- identify stressful situation
- deal with stress using various coping mechanisms

## MODULE 1 OUTLINE

| TOPICS | SUB-TOPICS TOTAL TIME 120 hours | LEARNING SITES/TIME | |
|---|---|---|---|
| | | Classroom 116 hours | One-on-One Assessment 2 hrs |
| Introduction 1.1 Personality Defined | * My assertive Self <br> *Personal Assessment [Assignment] <br> 1.1.1 Identification of Positive & Negative Traits <br> 1.1.2 Me & My Image Project (SICES PROFILE) | | |
| 1.2 Effective Communication | 1.2.1 Two Kinds of Communication <br> 1.2.2 Three Basic Interpersonal Needs <br> 1.2.3 Five Levels of Self-Disclosure <br> 1.2.4 Signs, Symbols and Ways of Communication <br> 1.2.5 Causes & Resolutions of Communication Breakdown <br><br> **INTERVIEW SCHEDULE:** <br><br> [**The Caregiver Application Form**] <br> **2 HRS** | | |
| 1.3 Coping Mechanism | 1.3.1 As a Process <br> 1.3.2 Common Stresses of a Caregiver | | |

TEXT: THE CAREGIVER RESOURCE MANUAL
Films on Canada by Duval Productions (CANADA & ITS PROVINCES)

**MODULE 2**

**Module 2**
**HEALTH AND SAFETY, FIRST AID & CPR**
**TOTAL ALLOTTED TIME - 120 HOURS**

TERMINAL OBJECTIVES OF MODULE 2

Upon completion of Module 2, the participant will be able to:
- qualify for certification to the Standard First Aid and Cardio-Pulmonary Resuscitation (CPR)
- recognize when first aid is needed
- give first aid at the scene of an accident/incident
- administer first aid at the scene of sudden illness
- prevent accidents and illnesses through the development of a health and safety oriented lifestyle
- recognize when more qualified help or medical help is required
- assist in giving medication
- safety proof the inside and outside of the house
- recognize & promote healing of various illnesses and diseases

MODULE 2 OUTLINE

| TOPICS | SUB-TOPICS TOTAL TIME 120 hours | | LEARNING SITES/TIME | |
|---|---|---|---|---|
| | | | Classroom 6 hours | One-on-One Assessment |
| 2.1 Introduction | 2.1.1 Terminologies<br>2.1.2 Responsibilities of the First Aider<br>2.1.3 The Emergency Scene Management | | | |
| 2.2 First Aid*<br>Classroom- 30 hrs<br>Workbook-6 hrs | 2.2.1 Artificial Respiration Unconsciousness<br>2.2.2 Choking<br>2.2.3 Wounds and Bleeding<br><br>2.2.4 Burns<br>2.2.5 Fractures and Joint Injuries | 2.2.6<br><br>2.2.7 Shock<br>2.2.8 Heat and Cold Injuries<br>2.2.9 Poisoning<br>2.2.10 Other Emergencies: Nose Bleeds/ Hypothermia/ Heat Stroke/ Bites.... | | 6 hours |
| 2.3 CPR* | 2.3.1 Infant/Child/Adult | | 24 hours | 6 hours |
| 2.4 Hazards | 2.4.1 Hazardous Product Symbols<br>2.4.2 Thermal Hazards<br>2.4.3 Electrical Hazards<br>2.4.4 Mechanical Hazards<br>2.4.5 Chemical Hazards | | 30 hours | |

| 2.5 Diseases | 2.5.1 Health & Safety Proofing the House<br>2.5.2 Communicable & Skin Diseases<br>2.5.3 Children's Diseases & Illness | 12 hours | |
|---|---|---|---|

TEXT: THE CAREGIVER RESOURCE MANUAL/St. John Standard Level Activity Book

First Aid & CPR Course Program provided by ST. JOHN AMBULANCE (Canada)

Films by St. John Ambulance

MODULE 3
A. HOME MANAGEMENT
TOTAL ALLOTTED TIME: 30 HOURS

TERMINAL OBJECTIVES OF MODULE 3 (Partial)

Upon completion of Module 3, the participant will be able to:
♦ define home and time management
♦ create a schedule of daily, weekly and monthly house chores
♦ identify various home appliances
♦ know how to use and maintain various home appliances

| TOPICS | SUB-TOPICS TOTAL TIME - 30 HRS | LEARNING SITES/TIME | | |
|---|---|---|---|---|
| | | Classroom 24 HRS. | Special Project Create a List of Chores & Schedule of Activities showing Daily, Weekly & Monthly House chores 6 hrs. | Critical Skills 8 HRS HOW TO: a. avoid litter using storage principles b. maintain and manage a home using a systematic approach *bedroom *living room *bathrooms *kitchen c. store food in the fridge/ freezer d. clean oven/ fridge/ cupboard |
| 3.1 Home Management | 3.1.1 Definitions 3.1.2 Checklist & Schedules | 1 hr. | | |
| 3.2 The Schedule of Activities | 3.2.1 Daily Routine 3.2.2 Weekly Schedule 3.2.3 Monthly Schedule 3.2.4 Assignment | 7 hrs. | | |
| 3.3 Home Appliances | 3.3.1 Uses 3.3.2 Maintenance 3.3.3 Energy Conservation 3.3.4 Individual Task Practice | 16 hrs | Practice using modern appliances | |

NOTES: *During the one-on-one assessment, the trainee must be able to verbally describe and explain the use of each of the major and small electrical appliances usually found in a home which include the vacuum cleaner, oven, stove, blender, fridge, washing machine, garborator, food processor, egg beater, clothes dryer, dishwasher, microwave oven, toaster, coffee maker, can opener. However, only the four major skills mentioned above are considered critical skills and each trainee must score 80% to pass. [In the event that the trainee scores less than 80%, he or she must schedule another assessment until the passing mark is achieved.]
*Participants are encouraged to use the centre to hone their skills on the use of the various electrical and major appliances with the use of the INDIVIDUALIZED TASK PRACTICE SHEETS.

**MODULE 3 B**

B. NUTRITION, BASIC FOOD PREPARATION & FOOD PRESENTATION
TOTAL ALLOTTED TIME - 90 HOURS

TERMINAL OBJECTIVES OF MODULE 3

Upon completion of Module 3, the participant will be able to:
♦ understand the concept and skills in handling food and prevent contamination
♦ understand the concept of nutrition and food preparation
♦ identify the four food groups and their alternatives
♦ know what nutrients are and their various functions and roles in the body.
♦ know basic cooking terminologies
♦ become familiar with North American cooking
♦ prepare and present North American dishes
♦ follow recipes

MODULE 3 OUTLINE

| TOPICS | SUB-TOPICS TOTAL TIME - 90 HRS | LEARNING SITES/TIME | | |
|---|---|---|---|---|
| | | Theoretical 30 HRS. | Lab 54 hrs | One-on-One 12 HRS |
| 4.1 The Four Food Groups | 4.1.1 Milk and Dairy Products    4.1.3 Bread & Cereal Group 4.1.2 Checklist & Schedules.    4.1.4 Fruits and Vegetables | | | |
| 4.2 Nutrients & Their Functions | 4.2.1 Basic Nutrients 4.2.2 Interlocking Patterns of Nutrients 4.2.3 Canada's Food Guide | 6 hrs. | | |
| 4.3 Basic Food Preparation/ Presentation | 4.3.1 Cooking Terminologies/ Recipes 4.3.2 Food Preparation/ Presentation *Breakfast*Lunch*Dinner/ Supper | 54 hrs (Lab) | Each group must plan, cook and serve a complete meal to a family.* | |
| 4.4 Special Project | 4.4.1 Collage Project: The Four Food Groups | | 6 hours | |

| 4.5 Food Management | 4.5.1 The Concept of Safe Food Handling<br>4.5.2 Prevention of Germs from Spreading<br>4.5.3 Food Contamination & Prevention | | 6 hours | |
| --- | --- | --- | --- | --- |

*Assessment Criteria: Food Guide, Food Appeal, Before and After Preparation
TEXT: THE CAREGIVER RESOURCE MANUAL: SICES PUBLICATION
Reference: Canada Food Guide, Health Canada Publication

**MODULE 4**

MODULE 4
CARE OF CHILD
TOTAL ALLOTTED TIME: 120 HOURS

TERMINAL OBJECTIVES OF MODULE 4
Upon completion of Module 3, the participant will be able to:
♦     state the philosophy of child care and identify the role of caregiver
♦     explain the importance of knowing child development needs and activities
♦     understand the concept of growth and child development
♦     plan to provide for the needs and activities of children
♦     describe the procedure for reporting child abuse
♦     apply the knowledge and skills gained through projects, presentations and independent study

| TOPICS | SUB-TOPICS TOTAL TIME - 120 hours | LEARNING SITES/TIMES (Classroom) | | |
|---|---|---|---|---|
| | | Theoretical | WORKBOOK FILMS: 4 hrs | *One-on-One Assessment 2 hrs |
| 5.1 Child Care<br><br>5.2 The Importance of Knowing Child Development | 5.1.1. Definition<br>5.1.2 SPICE as an Acronym Social/Physical/Intellectual/Creative/Emotional<br>5.2.1 Concepts of Growth and Development<br>5.2.2 Ages & Stages of Development<br>5.2.3 Basic Development Needs<br>5.2.4 Consequences when Needs are Not Met | 12 hours | Workbook<br>A. The Newborn<br>(0-1 year) | **HOW TO:**<br>**a. lift & hold a baby**<br><br>**b. bathe an infant**<br><br>**c. diaper a baby**<br><br>**d. prepare a formula**<br><br>**e. bottle feed a baby**<br><br>**f. burp a baby**<br><br>**g. dress up a baby**<br><br>**h. report a child abuse & when** |
| 5.3 SPICE Development | 5.3.1 Social Development<br>5.3.2 Physical Development<br>5.3.3 Intellectual Development<br>5.3.4 Creative Development<br>5.3.5 Provider or Emotional Activities | 12 hours | B. The Toddler<br>(1 -2 years)<br><br>C. The Preschooler<br>(2 - 5 years) | |
| 5.4 The Role of the Child Caregiver | 5.4.1 Provider of Social Activities<br>5.4.2 Provider of Physical Activities<br>5.4.3 Provider of Intellectual Activities<br>5.4.4 Creative Development<br>5.4.5 Provider of Emotional Activities | 12 hours | FILMS: 4 hrs.<br>1.Thinking Professionally<br>(30 mins). | |
| 5.5 Health & Safety | 5.5.1 Cleanliness/Sanitation<br>5.5.2 Personal Hygiene & Health<br>5.5.3 House Safety<br>5.5.4 Children 's Diseases | 12 hours | 2. Supporting Family Relations (30 mins) | |
| 5.6 The Value & Stages of Play | 5.6.1 The Value of Play<br>5.6.2 The Stages of Play<br>5.6.3 Toys & Play Equipment | 24 hours | 3.Communicating Through Children<br>(30 mins) | |
| 5.7 Child Abuse/ Management | 5.7.1 The Child Welfare Act of 1984<br>5.7.2 Child Management<br>5.7.3 Approaches to Child Management | 12 hours | 4. Facilitating Play<br>(30 mins) | |
| 5.8 Special Section | 5.8.1 Infant Care (How to: Bathe, Dress, Feed)<br>5.8.2 Nursery Rhymes<br>5.8.3 Games Children Play<br>5.8.4 Children's Favourite Stories<br>5.8.5 Role Playing/Skits/ Songs/Poems/ Stories | 30 hours | 5. Nurturing thru:<br>*social *physical<br>*creative and<br>*emotional<br>ACTIVITIES | |

*The trainee must obtain a passing mark of 80% on critical skills assessed or must repeat until passing mark is attained.
Text: The Caregiver Resource Manual

**MODULE 5**

MODULE 5

CARE OF THE SENIOR/Persons with Special Needs
TOTAL ALLOTED TIME - 120 HOURS

TERMINAL OBJECTIVES OF MODULE 5A

Upon completion of Module 5A, the participant will be able to:

♦    identify the three phases and types of aging
♦    describe the role of the caregiver
♦    appreciate the rights of the elderly
♦    understand the relationship between aging and nutrition
♦    recognize illness and disabilities due to aging
♦    know how to care for an elderly with disabilities
♦    perform personal and basic nursing care for the elderly
♦    apply knowledge and skills gained during class sessions

### MODULE 5A OUTLINE

| TOPICS | SUB-TOPICS TOTAL TIME - | LEARNING SITES/TIMES (Classroom) | | |
|---|---|---|---|---|
| | | Classroom & FILMS & Workbooks (114 hrs) | *One-on-One Assessment of Critical Skills 2 hrs | How to: 6 hours |
| 5.1 Three Phases of Aging | 5.1.1 The Pre-Retirement Phase 5.1.2 The Retirement Phase 5.1.3 The Post Retirement Phase | | | a. safe-proof the house b. wash hands and prevent germs from spreading c. feed a bedridden elderly |
| 5.2 Types of Aging | 5.2.1 Chronological Aging     6.2.3 Psychological Aging 5.2.2 Biological Aging     6.2.4 As a Companion | | | |
| 5.3 The Roles of the Caregiver | 5.3.1 As an Employee     6.3.3. As a Provider of Care 5.3.2 As a "Member" of the Family     6.3.4 As a Companion | | | d. exercise legs, hands, neck, body (deep breathing) |
| 5.4 Traits | 5.4.1 Case Studies Leading to the Identification of the Various       Characteristics of the Elderly Requiring Care | | | e.. effectively communicate f. arrange social & outdoor activities |
| 5.5 Needs and Activities | 5.5.1 The Importance of a Checklist of Needs and Activities 5.5.2 General Care     6.5.3 Personal & Nursing Care | | | g. arrange social visits to & from families & friends |
| 5.6 Aging and Nutrition | 5.6.1 Factors Affecting Nutrition 5.6.2 Food Groups & Nutrition | | | h. care for the feet |
| 5.7 Aging and Disabilities | 5.7.1 Aging & Disabilities | | | |

TEXT: THE CAREGIVER RESOURCE MANUAL

**MODULE 6**

MODULE 6
**SPECIAL PROJECT: MY FUTURE EMPLOYMENT**
**Total Allotted Time: 120 Hours**

TERMINAL OBJECTIVE OF MODULE 6:

Upon completion of Module 6, the participant will be able to:

- Have a thorough understanding of the community he or she will be living in.
- Describe in details and sketch the house of his or her future employer.
- Have a proposed or recommended Schedule of House Chores based on input from employer detailing daily, weekly and monthly chores.
- Provide a Month's Menu outlining Breakfast, Lunch , Supper including snacks.
- Have a complete profile of the person requiring care and a brief profile of the person's significant others.
- Provide a suggested Plan of Schedule of Activities
  For a child or children: Activities would reflect ages and stages of development
  For Persons with Special Needs: Activities would reflect SPICE capabilities.
- FOR PERSON WITH DISABILITY ONLY. Provide a review of literature on the ailments or disabilities of the person requiring care.
- Have a thorough understanding of the Rights and Freedom of the Caregiver while at work and on days off.
- Have a thorough understanding of the Live-in Caregiver Program and the caregiver's roles and legal responsibilities.

## MODULE 6 TOPIC OUTLINE

| TOPICS | SUB-TOPICS |
|---|---|
| 6.1 My Canadian Community<br>(18 hours) | 6.1.1 The Community<br>6.1.2 The Nearest City<br>6.1.3 The Province |
| 2.2  My Home in Canada<br>(18 hours) | 6.2.1 The Structure of the Home<br>2.2.2   The Appliances in the Home<br>2.2.3   Proposed Schedule of House Chores |
| 3.3   Menu Planning<br>(18 hours) | 3.3.1   The Family's Favourites<br>3.3.2   Proposed Menu for the Month<br>3.3.3   Recipes in Index Cards |
| 4.4   The Person I Will Care For<br>(18 hours) | 4.4.1   The Profile of the Person Requiring Care<br>4.4.2   SPICE Characteristics<br>4.4.3   Schedule of Special Needs/Activities<br>4.4.4   *Current Literature on Disability<br>[For Special Need Person Caregiver] |
| 4.5   The Caregiver Rights/Freedom<br>(18 hours) | 6.5.1 Review of Canada's Rights & Freedom<br>6.5.2 The Labor Laws of Canada<br>6.5.3The Provincial Labor Standards (Canada)<br>6.5.4 My Days Off |
| 4.6   The Live-in Caregiver Program<br>(18 hours) | 6.6.1 Questions and Answers |

*The above lessons will thoroughly familiarize the trainee with his or her future employer.

**Attempts should be made to regularly contact the employer through letters**

# MODULE
# 1
## Personality
## Effective Communication
## Work Values

# MODULE 1
## PERSONALITY ENHANCEMENT, CULTURAL ADAPTATION
## AND EFFECTIVE COMMUNICATION MODULE
## TIME ALLOTED - 120 HOURS

TERMINAL OBJECTIVES OF MODULE 1

Upon completion of Module 1, the participant will be able to:
- explain personality
- identify positive and negative personality traits
- create his own SPICE profile using assessment of self as well as feedback from significant others
- explain the acculturation process
- appreciate the impact of acculturation
- appreciate the HOST COUNTRY AND ITS PEOPLE
- appreciate CANADA, ITS GEOGRAPHY, FACTS AND FIGURES
- practise effective communication
- identify stressful situation
- deal with stress using various coping mechanisms

## MODULE 1 OUTLINE

| TOPICS | SUB-TOPICS TOTAL TIME 120 hours | LEARNING SITES/TIME | |
|---|---|---|---|
| | | Classroom 116 hours | One-on-One Assessment 2 hrs |
| Introduction 1.2 Personality Defined | * My assertive Self<br>*Personal Assessment [Assignment]<br>1.1.1 Identification of Positive & Negative Traits<br>1.1.2 Me & My Image Project (SICES PROFILE) | | |
| 1.2 Effective Communication | 1.2.1 Two Kinds of Communication<br>1.2.2 Three Basic Interpersonal Needs<br>1.2.3 Five Levels of Self-Disclosure<br>1.2.4 Signs, Symbols and Ways of Communication<br>1.2.5 Causes & Resolutions of Communication Breakdown<br><br>**INTERVIEW SCHEDULE:**<br><br>**[The Caregiver Application Form]**<br>**2 HRS** | | |
| 1.3 Coping Mechanism | 1.3.1 As a Process<br>1.3.2 Common Stresses of a Caregiver<br>1.3.3 Ways and Means of Handling Stress | | |

TEXT: THE CAREGIVER RESOURCE MANUAL
Films on Canada by Duval Productions (CANADA & ITS PROVINCES)

# CONTENTS OF MODULE 1

# 1.1 PERSONALITY ENHANCEMENT

## 1.1.1  MY ASSERTIVE SELF.

## My Assertive Self

**by Julie V. Kallal**

everything I do, think and say, there are aspects about me that I do not know or do not understand, therefore these aspects puzzle me. The fortunate thing is I am alive, therefore, I can find solutions to these puzzles and that's what's exciting about me. I am who I am at any given moment. If I looked back and reviewed what I said or did in the past or how I looked and felt in the past, it would only be because I wanted to reminisce and reflect on my experience and I would learn from it. What is important is now, my present looks, my present actions, my present state of mind. Tomorrow is an extension of today therefore, I can decide to plan and change my directions. But as I said before, my decisions are mine- I may rely on my own resourcefulness and do some thinking or researching, or I may decide to seek the help of professionals, friends, relatives or I may continue to be a life-long learner.

Hey, I know who I am and you know what? I'm o.k.? Are you?

Who am I?  In this world there is no one like me! I am unique!  There are others who approximate me, in terms of my looks, the way I dress or the way I talk. Ah! But they don't add up like me. Everything about me is mine alone – my body and everything it does- my speech, my actions, my feelings and my thinking, in short my behavior and ideas. I have my own dreams, ambitions, goals, fantasies, hopes, fears, successes, failures and errors. I think, therefore, I decide, choose, invent, create, solve problems, avoid conflicts, make mistakes, make plans, change plans and any other things that my mind can possibly think of. I can speak softly, loudly, angrily, cheerfully, aggressively, assertively or hatefully. Yes, I do enjoy the so called freedom of speech. I have feelings therefore I am capable of being in love, being angry, being jealous, being hurt, being frustrated, being disappointed, being excited, being moody or being happy. And am I also capable of hating, crying, smiling? You bet! Now, although I own myself and

## 1.1.2  PERSONAL ASSESSMENT PROJECT.

**ASSIGNMENT:**   Use a binder, a folder or a coiled notebook or a scrapbook to develop this assignment. You have to hand this in at the end of the module. You can also use a computer to answer the questions.

1. **How well do I know my vital statistics?**

Height/ weight/ chest/ waist/ hip/ shoe/ dress/ pant length

*Hint: Use own photo or cut-out from magazines.*

2. **If I were…**

| | | |
|---|---|---|
| a millionaire | an appliance | a precious stone |
| a building | a t.v. character | a plant |
| an animal | a book | a tree |
| an artist | a flower | a country |
| a car | a man/woman | a singer |
| an actor/actress | a computer | a house |

**I would…**

*Hint: If I were a millionaire, I would open a scholarship funds for the needy.*

3. **My favorite…**

| | | | | |
|---|---|---|---|---|
| color | perfume | song | actor | novel |
| sports | t.v. program | singer | actress | film |
| friend | relative | family member | one other | a person |

4. **What would I rather be… and why.**

| | | |
|---|---|---|
| wealthy | good looking | smart |
| a taxi | an elevator | a car wash |
| an artist | a musician | a dancer |
| a doorknob | a key | a window |
| a rainbow | a snowflake | a falling star |
| a snake | a lizard | a crocodile |

*Hint: Choose only one from across. Ex: Choose either wealthy, good looking or smart then develop your sentence.*

5. **Five (5) things that bug me… because (explain each one) …**

**6. Things I like to do...**

| | |
|---|---|
| that cost money | once in a while |
| with a friend | often |
| by myself | with my family |
| with someone I love | but can't |

*Hint: Develop each topic*

**7. My feelings...**

| | |
|---|---|
| I'm happy when... | I get excited when... |
| I get angry when... | I feel safe when |
| I hope that... | I need... |
| I'm good at... | I'm thankful for... |
| I'm afraid of... | I'm lonely when... |
| I'm ashamed of... | I'm proud of... |
| I feel sorry for... | I'm really good at... |

*Hint: Develop each topic.*

**8. My special message to the world...(an essay). Choose one or create your own.**

| | | | |
|---|---|---|---|
| Peace | War | Pollution | Abortion |
| Euthanasia | Crime | Violence | Charity |
| My Goals | Life | Education | The Future |
| Family | Values Drugs | | Poverty |

### 1.1.3  GETTING TO KNOW ME  (ME AND MY IMAGE).

**S**ocial                  how you relate with those around you
                          positively and negatively.

**P**hysical                your vital statistics; your physical activities such as
                          sports, hobbies; the food you like or dislike.

**I**ntellectual            activities that stimulate your mind such as reading
                          and discussions

**C**reative                activities that deal with your senses, hobbies.

**E**motional               the way you react to the world (total environment).

*Personality is the individual being – socially, physically, intellectually, creatively, and emotionally. It is the sum total of the individual's positive and negative traits.*

### ASSIGNMENT:

Make a creative poster describing yourself socially, physically, intellectually, creatively and emotionally.  This poster must incorporate how you and your significant others (your image) see you. Your image is how others see you. Your significant others may include your family, your friends, the people you work with, professionals you deal with (doctor, dentist, priest), people who do not particularly like you and any others who impact or influence you in your daily activities.

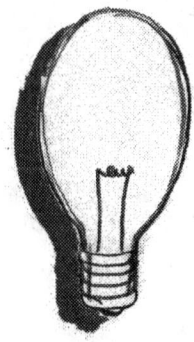

Helpful Tips:
Cut out pictures from magazines, draw, use actual photos
of you and your significant others. Use your imagination.

# 1.2 EFFECTIVE COMMUNICATION

## 1.2.1 BASIC VALUES THAT ENHANCE PERSONALITY.

There are four basic values that enhance personality:
a) Communication
b) Unity
c) Love
d) Forgiveness

## 1.2.2 TWO KINDS OF COMMUNICATION.

**Verbal** is communication that uses words. **Non-Verbal** is easy. It is a form of communication that does not use words; it is communication through physical behavior (i.e., body language, facial expressions, gestures, eye contact), vocal cues, and spatial relationships (distance/space between people).

Note: Research has found that whereas the verbal is responsible for conveying the cognitive and informational aspects of a message, the non-verbal conveys the affective or emotional aspects. In short:

*"It is not that I mind what is said but how it is said"*
*illustrates the role of the non-verbal communication.*

## 1.2.3 THREE BASIC INTERPERSONAL NEEDS (MOTIVATION TO COMMUNICATE).

| | |
|---|---|
| **Affection** | A person communicates to attain love from another human being and to know s/he can be loved. |
| **Inclusion** | A feeling of significance or importance. The need to belong |
| **Control** | The desire to feel responsible. It demonstrates competence in coping. |

### 1.2.4 FIVE LEVELS OF SELF-DISCLOSURE.

| Level | Type | Examples |
|---|---|---|
| 1 | **Senseless Conversation**<br>➢ Lowest level of communication<br>➢ An ice breaker | How are you?<br>What's happening?<br>It's nice to see you!<br>I'm glad you're here!<br>Let's have lunch sometime. |
| 2 | **Gossip Level**<br>➢ Reveals very little about one's self<br>➢ Talks about others instead | *Person 1:* You know what? I've seen Judy coming out of the hotel with Ferdie."<br>*Person 2:* Well, what do you know, I have been suspecting those two all along." |
| 3 | **My Idea/Opinion with No Sound Basis**<br><br>➢ Involves a little disclosure<br>➢ Some neutral information | Testing the other person's opinion.<br>*Person 1:* I think Judy and Ferdie are an item<br>*Person 2:* What made you think that? (Person 1 switches to Level 2 to carry on the gossip)<br>: No, they're just friends, believe me (Person 1 switches to Level 4 to gain acceptance) |
| 4 | **Self Conviction**<br>➢ True Feeling or Emotion<br>➢ Gut Feelings<br>➢ Involves revealing self-convictions | "As far as I'm concerned".<br>"I believe . . ."<br>"If you asked me . . ."<br>"The way I feel about it…"<br>"I really think that…" |
| 5 | **"Peek Level of Communication"**<br>➢ Deepest level<br>➢ Great trust on self | Instructor's Lectures<br>Church Sermons<br>Skills Demonstrations |

*Silence* is considered one of the most beautiful forms
of communication engaged in by the person.
It marks real meeting of the minds.

## 1.2.5  SIGNS, SYMBOLS AND WAYS OF COMMUNICATION.

### Ways of Communication:

| Verbal    -    Non-verbal  Vocal - Non-vocal | Speaking - Listening  Reading  - Writing |
|---|---|

### Statistics:

| Based on studies done on the way we communicate, the following indicates the percentages on how we communicate. | |
|---|---|
| 7% | Verbal |
| 38% | Vocal (Intonations and Voice Quality) |
| 55% | Facial Expressions |

## 1.2.6  CAUSES & RESOLUTIONS OF COMMUNICATION BREAKDOWN.

Causes of communication breakdown include"
- a)  Language Usage
- b)  Interpretation
- c)  Ineffective Listening
- d)  Ineffective Behavior
- e)  Ineffective Attitude
- f)  Action Language

## 1.2.7  RESOLUTIONS OF COMMUNICATION BREAKDOWN.

Examples of resolution are:
- a)  Confrontation
- b)  Not Speaking
- c)  Writing Notes
- d)  Arguing Back
- e)  Doing Nothing
- f)  Getting In A Fight
- g)  Walking Away
- h)  Discussion

## 1.2.8  THE INTERVIEW.

To have an effective interview, as a form of communication, the following are required:
- a)  The Purpose of the Interview – What is to be accomplished?
- b)  Background Information for the Interview

c) Preparation of Questions
d) The Importance of Careful Listening
e) The Importance of Note-Taking

| 1.3 | WORK VALUES |
|---|---|

## 1.3.1 THE COPING MECHANISM AS A PROCESS.

We all experience stress in varying degrees and in order to function effectively, we must attempt to cope with it. This coping takes place both at the conscious and unconscious levels and the capability of coping varies greatly from individual to individual.

Scientists state that in order to cope effectively, a balance must exist between the demands upon the individual and his capability for handling them. But why does the capability for handling stress vary so greatly between individuals? Howath (1978) suggests a theoretical view which sheds some light upon this question. In terms of preparation, he says, we have all come through four phases which to a large extent, determine our adjustment capabilities.

Each is a process as follows:

1. **Biological**
   In a primitive sense, each body has adapted itself along the way according to the needs. Thus, when the physical demands differ greatly from previous experience, the body has difficulty adapting.

2. **Developmental**
   During the stages of emotional development, a person's learning experiences have prepared him for a certain lifestyle. When radically different, emotional demands are imposed upon, the person has difficulty adapting.

3. **Social**
   During life, each individual acquires a variety of roles with which he gradually becomes comfortable. When he is forced to play unfamiliar or inconsistent roles, conflict is experienced and the pressure from that conflict, makes it progressively more difficult for the person to adapt.

4. **Phenomenological**
   Each individual develops a set of aspirations for his life goals to which he strives. When life experiences failure to match these expectations, frustration is experienced. Stress results, and the person finds it progressively more difficult to adapt.

All the foregoing describes our uniqueness in reacting to stress but it also implies our limitations. The situation, however, can be changed to some appreciable extent. It is possible for an individual to become aware of his coping mechanisms, recognize his limitations and develop new and positive ways of coping with stress.

## 1.3.2  COMMON STRESSES OF A CAREGIVER

| PHYSICAL | SOCIAL |
|---|---|
| • Excessive demands on physical strength<br>• Trying to handle work<br><br>• Biochemical changes previously described which would be activated of working in a new setting | • Demands from employer for more care<br>• Demands from caregiver's own family<br>• Being caught in the middle as "information-giver" among family members<br>• Negative professional self-concept |

There are still many other sources of stress that can be identified in each of the above categories which many times impact each other.

## 1.3.3  VARIOUS COPING MECHANISMS

### a) Communication
- One of the most effective ways of coping with stress or even preventing its occurrence is through effective communication.

### b) Self-Awareness
- It is important to become aware of the various activities that are stressful and why such activities can cause stress. Equally important is the effect that stress has on an individual mentally, physically and emotionally. By becoming aware, an individual can help himself to develop ways to manage stress more effectively.

## WAYS AND MEANS OF HANDLING STRESS
*(Source: The Canadian Mental Health Association)*

| Talk it out. | When something worries you, talk it out and sit down with somebody you trust your spouse, parent, friend, clergyman, family doctor, teacher or counselor. |
|---|---|
| Escape for a while. | It sometimes helps to escape from a problem for a short time. Read a book, go to a movie, go for a walk, go for a drive somewhere. It's not only therapeutic to escape punishment long enough to recover breath and balance but to be prepared to come back and look at the problem when you are more composed. |

| Give in occasionally. | If you find yourself getting into frequent quarrels and feeling defiant, remember that frustrated children behave the same way. Stand your ground but do it calmly and remember that you could be wrong. Even if you are sure you are right, it's sometimes easier to give in now and then. Have the satisfaction of hoping that the other person may someday realize his mistake and ask for your understanding. |
|---|---|
| Work off your anger. | While anger may give you temporary sense of righteousness, or even power, it will probably leave you feeling foolish. If you have the urge to lash out, wait a while, take a deep breath, deliberately postpone lashing out until tomorrow. Do something constructive with that pent-up energy instead – take a long walk, do your garden, shovel snow, clean up the basement. After a while, you'll be so absorbed that your anger is not as intense as before and before long, you face the problem in a much more civilized manner. |
| Take One Thing at a Time. | For people under tension, an ordinary workload may seem insurmountable. The task looks so large that it may become painful to tackle any part. Prioritize the tasks – do only a portion of it at a time. Do the biggest load first. Once the major task is done, the rest won't be so big any more. |
| Shun the "Superman" Role. | Some people expect too much of themselves. They strive for perfection in everything they do. The frustration of failure leaves them in a constant state of worry and anxiety. Decide what you do well and put your major effort into it. Once this is done, you will achieve a sense of success and satisfaction. Then you can tackle the ones that you can't do so well. Give it your best. It will not be so bad if at the end some tasks are not done the way they should have been done. You've given it your best – that's what counts. |
| Go Easy with Criticism. | Expecting too much of others can lead to feelings of frustration and disappointment. Each person has his own virtues, shortcomings, values . . . his own right to develop as an individual. Instead of being critical, search out the other's good points and help him to develop them. You'll find that after a while if you always try to at least look at the positive side of an individual, you'll like your new self and you will be less critical of others. |

# 1.4       MY DAILY JOURNAL

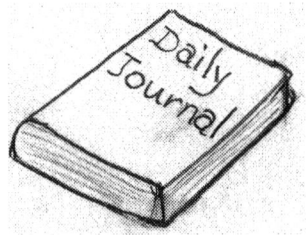

LCP Module 1: Personality Enhancement, Cultural Adaptation, Effective Communication and Q & A on the LCP Program

## INSTRUCTION:

In your daily journal, **WRITE EACH QUESTION FIRST, followed by your answers**. If the question is not written, the answers will not be considered by your instructor. You may answer the question in any order, but please indicate the question number for easy recording.

You have one full month to complete this work. Try to do one question a day, so you are always caught up.

1. Explain personality in your own words.

2. Using 2 columns, list your positive and negative personality traits.

3. Identify your strongest and weakest traits and justify them by giving some anecdotes or experiences relating to them.

4. Explain the stages of acculturation. If you are already in Canada, explain them as they relate to you.

5. Differentiate between the old and the new way of life in Canada.

6. Enumerate the Canadian Charter of Rights and Freedom.

7. List Canada's 10 provinces and 3 territories, their capitals and major cities on a chart.

8. Research using the Internet, 5 facts and information about the provinces and territories. You may solicit the help of your classmates who have access to the Internet.

9. State the three basic interpersonal needs and explain each.

10. Explain the importance of the five levels of self-disclosure. Which level of self-disclosure is involved in being teacher, a nurse, a caregiver, an actor and why.

11. Give the various, signs, symbols and ways of communication.

12. State the causes and resolutions of communication breakdown.

13. Identify the common stresses of a caregiver.

14. Identify your own stresses as a learner, a member of a family, a worker, a tourist, a dependent (Choose those that are applicable).

15. Describe the coping mechanisms discussed in your manual.

16. How do you cope with your own stresses?

17. Which of the coping mechanisms described in the book could you use?

18. Summarize what you have learned from this module. Include learning and skills from the lectures.

19. Write an essay on any of the following topics:

   * Effective Communication
   * My Ideal Self
   * My Ideal Role as a Caregiver

---

*This important activity plus the first 2 assignments (poster and personal assessment project) account to 40% of your total mark.*
*Again, you have until the end of the module or the month to complete it.*
***Good Luck!***

---

# MODULE
## 2
### Health and Safety
### First Aid and CPR

**MODULE 2**

## Module 2
## HEALTH AND SAFETY, FIRST AID & CPR
## TOTAL ALLOTTED TIME - 120 HOURS

TERMINAL OBJECTIVES OF MODULE 2

Upon completion of Module 2, the participant will be able to:
- qualify for certification to the Standard First Aid and Cardio-Pulmonary Resuscitation (CPR)
- recognize when first aid is needed
- give first aid at the scene of an accident/incident
- administer first aid at the scene of sudden illness
- prevent accidents and illnesses through the development of a health and safety oriented lifestyle
- recognize when more qualified help or medical help is required
- assist in giving medication
- safety proof the inside and outside of the house
- recognize & promote healing of various illnesses and diseases

### MODULE 2 OUTLINE

| TOPICS | SUB-TOPICS TOTAL TIME | LEARNING SITES/TIME | |
|---|---|---|---|
| | | Classroom 6 hours | One-on-One Assessment |
| 2.1 Introduction | 120 hours | | |
| | 2.1.1 Terminologies 2.1.2 Responsibilities of the First Aider 2.1.3 The Emergency Scene Management | | |
| 2.2 First Aid* Classroom-30 hrs Workbook-6 hrs | 2.2.1 Artificial Respiration 2.2.6 Unconsciousness 2.2.2 Choking 2.2.7 Shock 2.2.3 Wounds and Bleeding 2.2.8 Heat and Cold Injuries 2.2.4 Burns 2.2.9 Poisoning 2.2.5 Fractures and Joint Injuries 2.2.10 Other Emergencies Other Emergencies: Nose Bleeds/ Hypothermia/Heat Stroke/Bites.... | | 6 hours |
| 2.3 CPR* | 2.3.1 Infant/Child/Adult | 24 hours | 6 hours |
| 2.4 Hazards | 2.4.1 Hazardous Product Symbols 2.4.2 Thermal Hazards 2.4.3 Electrical Hazards 2.4.4 Mechanical Hazards 2.4.5 Chemical Hazards | 30 hours | |

| 2.5 Diseases | 2.5.1 Health & Safety Proofing the House<br>2.5.2 Communicable & Skin Diseases<br>2.5.3 Children's Diseases & Illness | 12 hours | |
|---|---|---|---|

TEXT: THE CAREGIVER RESOURCE MANUAL/St. John Standard Level Activity Book

First Aid & CPR Course Program provided by ST. JOHN AMBULANCE (Canada)

Films by St. John Ambulance

# CONTENTS OF MODULE 2

## 2.1                                INTRODUCTION

The Health and Safety covers the Emergency and Standard level course based on the complete guide to First Aid and Cardiopulmonary resuscitation (CPR) of St. John Ambulance. All the first aid and CPR courses are presented in a module format consisting of compulsory and elective lessons which include the medical condition and environmental illnesses and injuries.

It also explores the occupational health and safety and health policies; and the government's regulations and legislation in administering different procedures in assisting medicine administration. Included also are the legal implications, state health policies in assisting medicine administration.

The entire module is on skills development and enhancement. The lecture-demo of all First Aid and CPR techniques are on AUDIO VIDEO CASSETTES supplemented by live demo by instructors.

| 2.2 | ANATOMY AND PHYSIOLOGY |
|-----|------------------------|

## STRUCTURE AND FUNCTION OF THE HUMAN BODY

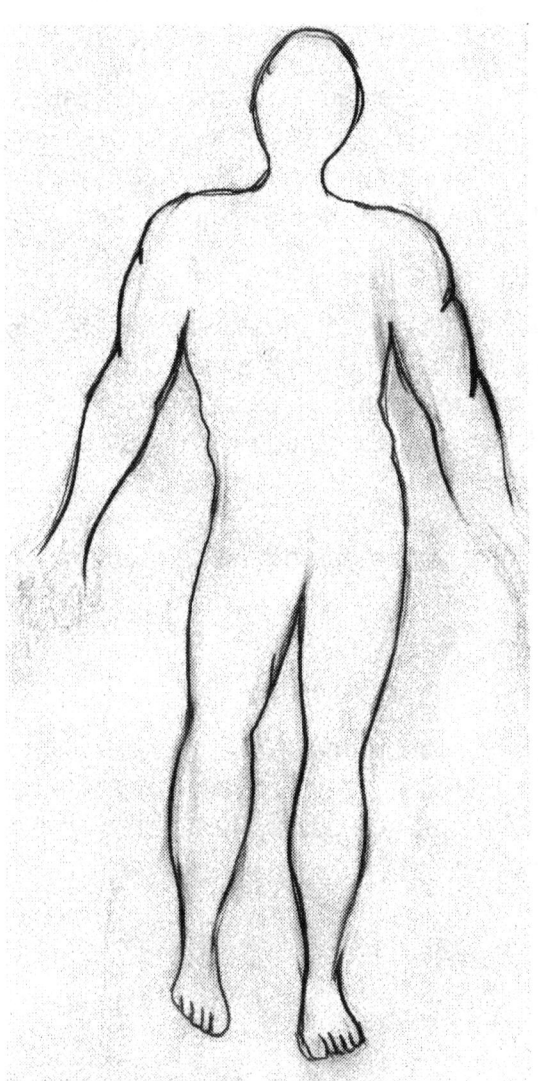

For one to administer first aid, intelligently, he should have some knowledge of the structure of the human body and the functions of its component parts. Basic information on human anatomy and physiology are included in order for the caregiver to have a knowledge base of the body, its systems, and their functions.

**Anatomy** is the study of the structure of the component parts of the body and their relationship to each other.

**Physiology** deals with the activity or functions of these various parts.

The main systems of the body are the circulatory, digestive, muscular, nervous, reproductive systems, respiratory, and skeletal systems.

### 2.2.1  CIRCULATORY SYSTEM

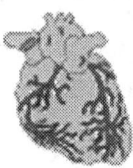

***The Heart.*** It is an organ about the size of a clenched fist. It pumps deoxygenated blood to the lungs, where carbon dioxide and oxygen exchange. Oxygenated blood returns to the lower part of the heart. This is known as ***the pulmonary circulation***.

***The systemic circulation*** carries the oxygenated blood and nutrition to all the other parts of the body, returning with the waste products that have to be filtered and excreted. Carbon dioxide is also returned to the heart by the systemic circulatory system, where after being pumped through the heart chambers, it enters the pulmonary circulatory system, and so the process starts again. Artery carries the oxygenated blood to all parts of the body while the veins pick up the deoxygenated blood and return it to the heart and lungs for another purification or oxygination.

## 2.2.2 DIGESTIVE SYSTEM

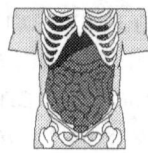 ***Digestion*** starts in the mouth. Food is chewed and mixed with saliva, which contains enzymes that make a start on the process of breaking larger molecules down into smaller ones which are more easily absorbed. The saliva also lubricates the food, making it softer and easier to swallow.

The ingested food then enters the esophagus and travels to the stomach. Here it is churned and mixed together with the stomach acids that change the food substances into a state that is more easily absorbed. The mixture then enters the small intestine and the large intestine, where further breakdown and absorption take places. The unabsorbed residue is expelled through the rectum and anus.

The liver, gall bladder, and pancreas are also important in the digestion process.

## 2.2.3 MUSCULAR SYSTEM

Muscles are composed of tissues which can be contracted so that movement can occur. They convert energy from food and respiration into physical movement, usually in response to signals from the brain and nervous system. They make up 35 to 45 percent of the average person's weight.

### 3 Types of Muscle Tissues:

There are three main types of muscle tissues:

***Skeletal.*** This type of muscle tissue is under the mind's conscious control, and it will respond to nervous signals by controlling the movement of the relevant bone (for example, the biceps pulls on the humerus to elevate the upper arm). There are over 650 skeletal muscles throughout the body.

***Smooth.*** This is found in the intestines and the linings of organs, and is not under conscious control.

**Cardiac.** This is a special type of involuntary tissue and is found only in the heart.

## 2.2.4  NERVOUS SYSTEM

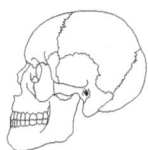

The nervous system is made up of 2 parts: Central Nervous System and Peripheral Nervous System.

***Central Nervous System.*** It consists of the brain and spinal cord.

***Peripheral Nervous System.*** It carries information from various parts of the body, through the relevant sensory nerves to the central nervous system. It carries out instructions through the efferent motor nerves (nerve cells which carry impulses away from the central nervous system related parts of the body). The nerves are made up of thousands of long thin nerve fibres. All the body systems consist of different types of cells.

## 2.2.5  REPRODUCTIVE  SYSTEM

***Male Reproductive System.*** Most of the male reproductive anatomy is external. The two testes hang in scrotal sacs. Two long convuluted tubes called the epididymis, one on each side, are attached to the testes. These allow the sperm which have been produced in the testes to ripen. The epididymis then opens into the vas deferens, another two long tubes – one on each side of the body – which are joined to the seminal vesicles. The seminal vesicle acts as a storage place mature sperm before they are released through the centre of the prostate gland and the urethra.

***Female Reproductive System.*** The female reproductive organ consists of the ovaries, fallopian tubes, uterus, and breasts.

The testes and ovaries produce reproductive cells that are called spermatozoa and ova. They also produce hormones that influenced body development and behaviour.

## 2.2.6  RESPIRATORY SYSTEM

The human respiratory system is made up of the nose and mouth, the pharynx and the larynx in the throat, and the windpipe or trachea then divides into two bronchi, which enter the lungs. The bronchi subdivide into smaller bronchioles, and they in turn subdivide into the alveolar ducts of the alveolar sacs, which contain the individual alveoli. The main muscles used in breathing are the intercostal muscles (these run between the ribs   and   the diaphragm).

***Respiration*** in human is the process by which oxygen is converted during metabolism to produce carbon dioxide. This gaseous exchange occurs through the alveoli in the lungs.

## 2.2.7  SKELETAL SYSTEM

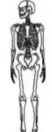 The bones give the body support and protect the internal glands and organs. They also give the body its shape, and they regulate minerals, particularly calcium phosphorus, copper and cobalt.  Healthy bone marrow is vital, as it manufactures red and white blood as well as platelet cells.

| 2.3 | FIRST AID |
|-----|-----------|

### 2.3.1  IMPORTANT TERMS

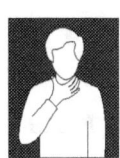

| **Artificial Respiration** | Is simply breathing for the casualty by providing appropriate breath. |
|---|---|
| **Casualty** | A person who is injured or who suddenly becomes ill. |
| **Choking** | A person chokes when the airway is partly or completely blocked and airflow is reduced or cut off. A choking person may die if first aid is not given immediately. |
| **CPR** | Cardio-Pulmonary Resuscitation. |
| **Fainting** | A brief of loss of consciousness caused by a temporary shortage of oxygen to the brain. |
| **First Aid** | The emergency help given to an injured or suddenly ill person using readily available materials. |
| **First Aider** | Someone who takes charge of an emergency scene and gives first aid. |
| **Medical Help** | The treatment given by, or under the supervision of, a medical doctor at an emergency scene, while transporting a casualty, or at a medical facility. |
| **The Emergency Scene Management (ESM))** | The sequence of actions you should follow at the scene of an emergency to ensure that safe and appropriate first aid is given.<br><br>The ESM has four steps, they are:<br>1.  Scene survey<br>2.  Primary survey<br>3.  Secondary Survey<br>4.  Ongoing casualty care until hand over |
| **Shock** | A condition of inadequate circulation to the body tissues. It results when the brain and other vital organs are deprived of oxygen. The development of shock can be gradual or rapid. It is a major emergency. It can accompany severe injury, emotional trauma, extensive infection, heart attack and any kind of accidents or injury. The casualty is pale, his skin cold and clammy, his breathing quick and irregular and his pulse is fast. |

### 2.3.2  AGE GUIDELINES FOR A CASUALTY

For first aid and CPR techniques, a casualty is considered to be:

- **An Adult**   :   8 years of age and over
- **A Child**    :   1 to 8 years of age
- **An Infant**  :   under 1 year of age

Note: Use these guidelines with common sense in choosing the appropriate first aid and CPR techniques. Consider the size of each casualty when making your decision.

### 2.3.3  THE RESPONSIBILITIES OF A FIRST AIDER

1. Assess the situation.
2. Determine quickly what assistance is needed to be given.
3. Assess the condition of the injured or ill person.
4. Establish priorities for care and give appropriate first aid.
5. Do the necessary report either to the proper authorities or parents.

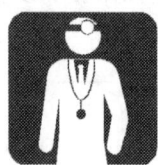

### 2.3.4  OBJECTIVES OF FIRST AID

- ➢ Preserve life
- ➢ Prevent the injury or illness from becoming worse
- ➢ Promote recovery.

### 2.3.5  3 PRIORITIES OF FIRST AID:

**Airway**
**Breathing**
**Circulation**

## 2.3.6  FIRST AID TREATMENT FOR SOME COMMON INJURIES/ILLNESSES

| Injury / Illness | Definition / First Aid |
|---|---|
| 1.    **Ear ache** | Immediate treatment requires diagnosis of the underlying cause. Always consult your doctor. For temporary relief, lie down and elevate the head using several pillows. Place a hot pad or hot water bottle over the ear and side of the head. Do not blow your nose. Avoid the use of ear drops unless prescribed by a doctor. Chewing gum may sometimes relieve the pain. |
| 2.    **Nose bleed** | Pinch the nostril just below bony bridge of nose. Hold tight (apply pressure) for at least 10 minutes or until blood clot forms. Casualty may lean forward (never backward). |

| | |
|---|---|
| **3.    Poisoning**<br><br>*Phone Numbers:*_____<br>_____<br><br><br>*Poison Centre:*_____<br>_____<br><br><br><br>*Doctor  :*_____<br>_____<br><br><br><br>*Type of Poison Treatment:*<br>_____<br>_____ | ➤    **Inhaled Poison:**<br>1.  Remove casualty to fresh air<br>2.  Apply artificial respiration, if required.<br>3.  Keep casualty warm. |
| | ➤    **Swallowed Poison (general ):**<br>If the person is conscious and able to swallow, immediately dilute the poison by giving the casualty 2 to 4 cups of milk or water. |
| | ➤    **Swallowed Poison (corrosives):**<br>*Ex: Gasoline, drain cleaners, oven cleaners,    turpentine,    bleach, kerosene*<br><br>1.  **DO NOT INDUCE VOMITING.**<br>2.  Give milk or water. If vomiting occurs naturally, hold head below hips to avoid choking. |
| | ➤    **Absorbed Poison (skin or eyes):**<br>1.  Flood the affected area with water.<br>2.  Remove contaminated clothing.<br>3.  **DO NOT ATTEMPT TO USE CHEMICAL ANTIDOTE.** |
| | ➤  **For All Substances Not Listed Above:**<br>1.  **INDUCE VOMITING.**<br>2.  Have casualty drink 2 to 4 glasses of milk or water. |

| | | |
|---|---|---|
| 4. | **Severe Bleeding** | A wound is any break in the continuity of the soft tissues of the body.<br><br>Types of Bleeding<br>1. **Arterial Bleeding.** Bleeding from an artery is characterized by a pulsating flow of bright red blood which usually accumulates rapidly. If this occurs from deep within a wound, pulsation may be absent but the volume is large and the color is bright red and spurts with each heart beat from the damaged artery. Arterial bleeding is serious and often hard to control.<br>2. **Venous Bleeding.** Venous blood is dark red in color and flows with a steady slow stream without pulsation. If venous bleeding occurs in an arm or leg, elevation of that extremity with slow the flow. Then pressure with the hand over a gauze compress, if one is available, will permit a clot to form. This pressure, for a minimum of two minutes and preferably for five minutes, is usually adequate. If bleeding continues, a tight compression bandage is applied.<br>3. **Capillary Bleeding.** A slow ooze as from a porous surface characterizes capillary bleeding. This is most frequent in a superficial injury resembling an abrasion or scraped area. A sterile bandage or, if none is present, a freshly ironed towel or pillow case placed over the wound and then secured with a bandage or hand pressure for several minutes usually suffices. In the occasional patient with a blood clotting defect, bleeding will continue but capillary oozing is usually not |

| 5. | **Swelling and Pain** | To minimize swelling, elevate and apply cold compresses. Cold helps contract blood vessels and tends to reduce swelling and pain. |
|---|---|---|
| 6. | **Toothache** | If toothache is the result of a cavity, clean the tooth with a cotton swab, then pack the tooth with a bit of sterile cotton soaked with an anaesthetic . If the pain is in some part of the jaw or gum, apply ice pack or hot water bottle to the face where the pain is located. Aspirin may help relieve the pain temporarily. See a dentist as soon as possible. |
| 7. | **Unconsciousness** | Loss of unconsciousness may threaten life if a person is on the back and the tongue has dropped to the back of the throat, blocking the airway. *To do:* 1. Make certain the person is breathing, then turn into the recovery position. 2. Never give anything by mouth to an unconscious casualty. 3. Get medical help and check breathing frequently. |

## 2.3.7 HAZARDS

### 4 Types of Hazards

➢ **Thermal or heat**

➢ **Chemical**

➢ **Mechanical**

➢ **Electrical**

### Hazardous Products

➢ Poison

➢ Explosive

➢ Radiation

➢ Flammable

### Severity of Hazards

➢ Caution

➢ Warning

➢ Danger

| | | | |
|---|---|---|---|
| 2-9 | 2-10 | 2-11 | 2-12 |
| 2-13 | 2-14 | 2-15 | 2-16 |

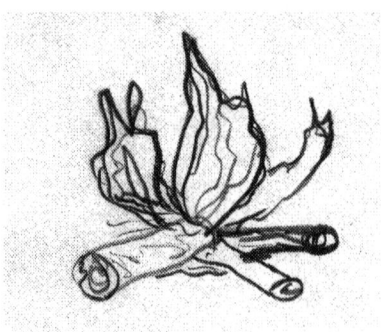

# 1.) THERMAL (HEAT) HAZARDS

**Sources of heat hazards :**
fireplaces, kitchen ranges and ovens, hot water, irons, flammable liquids, outdoor barbecues, matches and lighters

**To hazard proof, use the following checklist:**
_____1.   Keep matches and lighters out of reach of children.
_____2. Point pot handles toward the back of the stove.
_____3. Keep fire extinguisher handy and up to date.
_____4. Check smoke alarm equipment and replace batteries when necessary.
_____5. Store  flammable liquids in a safe place.
_____6. Keep drapes away from stove.
_____7. Be careful when turning on hot water tap.
_____8 Unplug flat iron when not in use.

## 2.)   CHEMICAL HAZARDS

**Sources of chemical hazards:**   Many products contain chemicals that may be toxic if swallowed, breathed or absorbed. Some may be corrosive, flammable or irritable to the skin and eyes. Examples are drugs, household cleaners, flammable liquids, aerosols, insecticides, bleaches and gas stoves.

**Use the checklist below often:**
_____1.   Always read the label of containers.
_____2.   Do not transfer any chemicals from the original containers into bottles & food containers.
_____3.   Keep cleaning products, medicines and cooking products away from children.
_____4.   Store chemicals properly. Do not store cooking and cleaning chemicals in the same place.
_____5.   Check gas ranges and barbecues often for leaks.
_____6.   Use gloves when handling corrosive products.
_____7.   Turn off gas regulators after each use.
_____8.   Avoid eating or drinking food that contain hazardous chemicals.
_____9.   Know your house plants and avoid keeping poisonous ones.
_____10. Never take medicines in the dark.
_____11. Dispose expired medicines and canned goods.

### 3.)    *MECHANICAL HAZARDS*

_____1.  Keep all power appliances and cutting machines in good repair.
_____2.  Avoid putting movable rugs on floors.
_____3.  Place gate at the top of stairs if there are children at home.
_____4.  Keep sturdy handrails along the wall down the stairs.
_____5.  Always check playground equipment and repair.
_____6.  Always check children's toys and discard broken ones.
_____7.  Use safety glasses when using saws and electrical equipment that produce sparks.
_____8.  Glass doors and walls should be marked with some kind of decals so that people can see from both directions.

### 4.)    *ELECTRICAL HAZARDS*

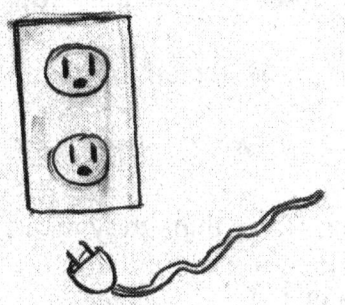

**Sources of electrical hazards:** Overloaded circuits can cause electrical fire. Other sources include extension cord and wall sockets, electric saws, drills, toaster, hair dryers, electrical appliances and faulty house wiring.

**The following can serve as a checklist to prevent electrical hazards:**

_____1.  Do not overload electrical outlets, extension cords and circuits.
_____2.  Know how to disconnect the main power source in the house.
_____3.  Be sure electrical appliances are properly grounded.
_____4.  Keep electrical appliances out of the bathroom.
_____5.  Prevent electrical cords from crossing hall ways.
_____6.  Use dummy plugs on outlets to keep children from getting shocked.
_____7.  Repair appliance cords and faulty appliances.

## 2.4                         DISEASES

### 2.4.1   HOW TO PREVENT GERMS FROM SPREADING

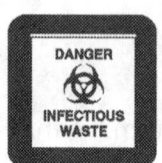

Germs thrive in warm, moist, and dark conditions. They are capable of surviving outside their natural environment for a period of time. The transmission of germs into the body can be direct or indirect. Disease causing germs can enter the body through the nose, mouth, ears, eyes, cuts, rectum, vagina and wounds.

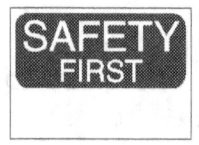

a. **Direct Contact.** Transmission of germs through direct contact can occur through physical contact.
   *Ex: touching or inhaling while a person sneezes*

b. **Indirect Contact.** Indirect contact however, occurs through the use of contaminated articles.
   *Ex: Use of dirty utensils, glasses or soiled cloth or bandages*

### 2.4.2   UNIVERSAL PRECAUTIONS TO CONTROL SPREAD OF DISEASE

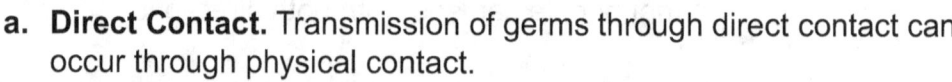

Some people are afraid to give first aid. They think they might catch a disease from the casualty. The risk of a serious infection being transmitted when giving first aid is small. Use the following universal precautions to minimize this risk and give first aid safely.

**Some simple ways of controlling the spread of germs:**
1. Avoid direct contact with persons with infectious diseases.
2. The mouth/nose should always be covered when coughing or sneezing.
3. Glasses, dishes and cutlery of the ill person should be washed immediately after use.
4. Wash hand thoroughly before and after attending to the ill person.
5. Wear vinyl or latex gloves whenever you might be in touch with the casualty's blood, body fluids, open wounds or sores.
6. Handle sharp objects with extra care.
7. Minimize mouth to mouth contact during artificial respiration by using a mask or a face shield designed to prevent disease transmission.

### BE IMMUNIZED.

### COVER A SNEEZE.

### WASH BEFORE EATING

### WASH HANDS AFTER USING TOILET.

## 2.4.3  MEDICAL CONDITION

| | |
|---|---|
| **Allergic reaction** | The response of body with an abnormal sensitivity to substances that are normally harmless. |
| **Bronchial Asthma** | Involves repeated attacks of shortness of breath with wheezing and coughing. |
| **Convulsion** | An infant or young child with a rapid rise in body temperature to $40^0$F is at risk of convulsions. A fever emergency is when the temperature taken in the armpit is $38^0$C ($100.5^0$F) or higher for an infant and $40^0$C ($104^0$F) higher for a child. |
| **Dehydration** | Drying out of the body loss of more water than taken in. Dehydration may be induced for medical reasons, but often it is an aspect of disease or injury, characterized by dry mucous membranes, fever, scanty urine, tight abdominal skin, possible shock. Treatment requires recognition of underlying circumstances, replacement of water and salts (sometimes plasma or blood) by infusion into the veins. |
| **Diabetes** | A condition in which the body does not produce enough insulin, causing the sugar level to be out of balance. |
| **Epilepsy** | A disorder of the nervous system |
| **Frostbite** | Exposure to extreme cold which cause a local tissue damage. |
| **Heat cramps** | Painful muscle spasms caused by an excessive loss of salt and water during sweating. |
| **Heat exhaustion** | Occurs when excessive sweating causes a loss of  body fluids and when a hot environment and high humidity do not allow the body to cool by sweating. |
| **Hypertension** | Abnormally high arterial blood pressure. |
| **Hypothermia** | A generalized cooling of the  body with body temperature falling below $35^0$C ($95^0$F). It usually develops from exposure to abnormally low temperatures over a prolonged period of time. |

## 2.4.4  MEDICINE ADMINISTRATION

R<sub>x</sub>

| | | |
|---|---|---|
| **Pharmacy** | : | The science and art of preparing drugs and forming them into suitable compounds for dispensing. |
| **Pharmacology:** | | The theory of pharmacy that looks at the action of drugs. |

| Variables that influence the drug action in the body | |
|---|---|
| Age<br>Administration Time<br>Body Weight<br>Chemical make-up of drugs<br>Compliance<br>Environment<br>Food/Medication | Genetics<br>Illnesses/Diseases<br>Interactions with other drugs<br>Level of Activity<br>Psychological Factors<br>Sex |

**2-21**

## 2.4.5  DRUG CLASSIFICATION

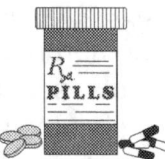

| | |
|---|---|
| Antibiotics | Anti-spasmodic |
| Anti-coagulants | Cardiac |
| Anti-convulsants | Depressants |
| Anti-hypertensive | Diuretics |
| Anti-inflammatory | Narcotics |
| Anti-psychotics | Stimulants |

## 2.4.6  CLIENT RIGHTS REGARDING MEDICATIONS:

1. To be informed of drug name, purpose, action and potential side effects (usually the responsibility of the physician, pharmacist or registered nurse)
2. To refuse a medication – regardless of the consequences.

| 2.5 | HOME SAFETY |
|-----|-------------|

## 2.5.1  SAFE-PROOFING YOUR HOME

There are five easy steps to exercise when safety-proofing your home.
1. Know the hazards,
2. Take the necessary precautions.
3. Be constantly alert.
4. Have a  list of emergency phone numbers near your phone and
5. Make sure you have a well stocked first aid in a handy place in your home.

## 2.5.2  HOME ACCIDENTS

a.  **Falls.** Fatal falls account 42% of the home accident death total, and about 8 out of every 10 occur in the 65 and over age group.

*Causes for Falls.* There are variety of reasons, such as falls from    ladders or scaffolding, falls from slipping, tumbling or tripping and    falls from pushing or shoving by or with another person.

*Reminders:*
1.  Never use a chair or a box in place of a sturdy ladder.
2.   When you use a ladder make sure it is in good condition before you trust it with your life.
3.  Don't have electric lamp cord trailing across the floor.
4.  Have additional base plugs installed so long cords are not necessary.

b.  **Fire, Burns, Scalds.** The second highest fatal accident in homes is fire, burns and scalds. Children under the age of 15 historically account for about 20% of the victims. The greatest cause of fire deaths involving children results from leaving them alone in the home.

*Reminders:*
1.  Don't leave children unattended- even for just a few minutes. Fire can start quickly and may prevent you from rescuing the youngsters.
2.  Never put a cigarette on a counter or any place except a deep ashtray and never smoke in bed.
3.  Don't dump ashtrays of cigarette stubs into a wastebasket or garbage bag. Cigarette stubs should be immersed in water before they are discarded.
4.  Supervise children around bonfires.

**2-22**

**_Burns_** are the leading cause of injury in the home, particularly among elderly people and young children. See the St. John Manual for details.

**_Scalds_** resulting from hot top water are on the rise. You can avoid this by adjusting the thermostat on your water heater to no higher than $54^0$ C ($130^0$ F). Be aware that even at this temperature, third degree burns can occur within 30 seconds. Never let children play near hot water.

**_Firearms_** every year, more than 60 Canadian die in firearms accidents, with about one quarter of these occurring in the home. Most victims are in the 15 to 34 age group.

| 2.6 | EMERGENCY SCENE MANAGEMENT |
|---|---|

### 2.6.1  FIRST AID.

First aid is the emergency help given to an injured or suddenly ill person using readily available materials.

### 2.6.2  OBJECTIVES OF FIRST AID.

The objectives of first aid are the following:
- To preserve life.
- To prevent the injury or illness from becoming worse.
- To promote recovery.

### 2.6.3  A FIRST AIDER.

A first aider is someone who takes charge of an emergency scene and gives first aid. A first aider has a First Aid Certificate.

### 2.6.4  AS A FIRST AIDER.

As a first aider, you can help a person in need.  The principles of the Good Samaritan Laws will protect you, as you:

- Act in good faith and volunteer your help.
- Tell the person you are a first aider.
- Get permission (consent) to give first aid before touching the casualty. Use your common sense; consider the age and the condition of the casualty.
- Ask the parents or guardian for permission if the person is an infant or young child.
- Have implied consent.  If the person does not respond to you, you can give first aid.  Implied consent exists because the casualty is unconscious and does not object to your help.
- Use reasonable skill and care according to your level of training.  Give the care you would like to get if you were in the casualty's position.
- Do not abandon (leave) the person once your offer of help has been accepted.

### 2.6.5  MEDICAL HELP

Medical help is the treatment given by, or under the supervision of, a medical doctor at an emergency scene, while transporting a casualty, or at a medical facility.

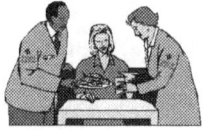

## 2.6.6  THE CASUALTY

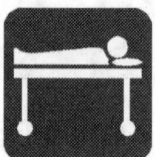

A person who is injured or who suddenly becomes ill is called a casualty.

## 2.6.7  AGE GUIDELINES FOR A CASUALTY

For first aid and CPR techniques, a casualty is considered to be:

- An adult – eight years of age and over
- A child – from one to eight years of age
- An infant – one year of age

## 2.6.8  UNIVERSAL PRECAUTIONS IN FIRST AID

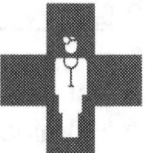

Some people are afraid to give first aid.  They think they might catch a disease from the casualty.  The risk of a serious infection being transmitted when giving first aid is small.  Use the following universal precautions to minimize this risk and give first aid safely.

- Wash your hand with soap and running water immediately after any contact with casualty.
- Wear vinyl or latex gloves whenever you might be touch with the casualty's blood, body fluids, open wounds sores.
- Handle sharp objects with extra care.
- Minimize mouth-to-mouth contact during artificial respiration by using a mask or a face shield designed to prevent disease transmission.

A face mask or face shield should:

- Have a one-way valve.
- Be disposable or have a disposable valve.
- Be stored in an easily accessible place.

## 2.6.9  PRINCIPLES OF EMERGENCY SCENE MANAGEMENT (ESM)

### *EMERGENCY SCENE MANAGEMENT (ESM)*

ESM is the sequence of action you should follow at the scene of an emergency to ensure that safe and appropriate first aid is given.

The order of the steps in ESM, including the priorities of first aid, may change, depending on the circumstances.

**STEPS IN ESM**

The ESM has 4 steps, usually in this order:

| |
|---|
| 1.  Scene survey. |
| 2.  Primary survey. |
| 3.  Secondary survey (taught as an elective lesion). *This step may not need to be done if first aid for life threatening conditions has been given and medical help is on the way.* |
| 4.  On going casualty care until hand over. |

### 1.)     Scene survey

The order of steps in the scene survey may change, but in most cases, you will do them in this order:

a.  Take charge of the situation.  If head/spinal injuries are suspected, tell casualty no to move.
b.  Call for help to attract bystanders
c.  Assess hazards at the scene and make the area safe for yourself and others
d.  Determine the number of casualties, what happened and the mechanism of injury for each
e.  Identify yourself as a first aider.  Offer to help and obtain consent.
f.  If head/spinal injuries are suspected, do not move the casualty. Provide and maintain manual support for head and neck.
g.  Assess the casualty the casualty's responsiveness.  If the casualty is not responsive, send or go for medical help.

### 2.)     Primary survey.

The primary survey is the first step in assessing the casualty for life threatening conditions and giving life-saving first aid.

In the primary survey you check for the priorities of first aid.  These are:

| A | - | **Airway** | To ensure a clear airway |
|---|---|---|---|
| B | - | **Breathing** | To ensure effective breathing |
| C | | **Circulation** | To ensure effective circulation |
| - | | | |

Even if there is more than one casualty, you should perform a primary survey on each casualty in turn.  Give life-saving first aid only.

### 3.)    Secondary survey.

The secondary survey is a step by step gathering of information which will help you to get a complete picture of the condition of the casualty.

The secondary survey consists of four steps that you should do in the following order:

- a.   Obtain the history of the casualty
- b.   Assess and record vital signs
- c.   Perform a head-to-toe examination

#### *History of the casualty*

By taking the history of a casualty, you are trying to find out everything that is important about the casualty's condition. A simple way to ensure that you take a complete history of the casualty, is to remember the word SAMPLE, where each letter stands for a part of the history:

| | |
|---|---|
| **S** = | Symptoms |
| **A** = | Allergies |
| **M** = | Medications |
| **P** = | Past and present medical history |
| **L** = | Last meal |
| **E** = | Event leading to the incident |

- Ask the conscious casualty how she feels now.  Be guided by the casualty's complaints
- If the casualty is unconscious, ask relative or bystanders about the casualty and the situation

#### *Vital signs*

The vital signs are important indicators of a casualty's condition.  The four vital signs you will learn about are:

- a.  Level of consciousness
- b.  Breathing
- c.  Pulse
- d.  Skin condition

## 4.)   Ongoing Casualty Care Until Hand Over.

Following immediate first aid, you must maintain the casualty in the best possible condition until hand over to medical help.

a.  Instruct a bystander to maintain manual support of the head and neck, if head/spinal injuries are suspected.
b.  Continue to steady and support any injuries are manually, if needed.
c.  Give first aid for shock.
   - Reassure the casualty often.
   - Loosen tight clothing.
   - Place the casualty in the best position for her injury or illness.
   - Cover the casualty to preserve body heat.

d.  Monitor the casualty's condition (ABC's) and note any changes
e.  Give nothing by mouth
f.  Record the casualty's condition, any changes that may occur and the first aid given
g.  Protect the casualty's personal belongings
h.  Do not leave the casualty until medical help takes over
i.  Hand over medical help and report on the incident, the casualty's condition and the first aid given.

## 2.7                           QUESTIONS

1. What will you do if you and your child are trapped inside a burning house?

2. What will you do if the complete airway obstruction casualty is pregnant or very obese?

3. What are the some important characteristics a first aider should possess?

4. What is the importance of knowing the Anatomy and Physiology in First Aid Training?

5. What is the first aid for choking-adult?

6. What is a fracture?

7. What is the first aid for first degree burn?

8. How will you give Artificial Respiration (AR) to a casualty who is wearing dentures?

9. As a first aider, how do you safeguard yourself?

10. How do you prevent choking among young children?

11. What will be your first aid when a child is suffering from earache?

12. What is an Emergency Scene Management (ESM)?

13. How will you give artificial respiration to a casualty with neck fracture?

14. What is a wound?

15. What is a sprain?

16. What are the 3 objectives of first aid?

17. What would you do if you suspect that a person is having a heart attack?

18. How do you prevent a shock from becoming worse?

19. What is the first aid for convulsion in young children?

20. What is artificial respiration (AR)?

21. What are the responsibilities of a first aider?

22. What will you do if the middle of your administration of CPR to a casualty, he/she vomits?

23. What will you do when a conscious choking casualty becomes unconscious?

24. What is muscle strain?

25. How do you keep the child safe in the house?

26. What is a poison?

27. What are the 2 types of poisons and the corresponding first aid for each?

28. What is an illness?

29. What is First Aid?

30. If the child falls, gets bumps/ bruises, and swelling develops rapidly, how do you manage the situation?

31. What are the signs of shock?

32. What will you do if a child is suffering from a toothache?

33. How do you give CPR to an adult?

34. What are the differences in giving cardio-pulmonary resuscitation (CPR) to a child and an infant?

35. What is the first aid for a person about to faint?

36. How do you prevent colic?

37. What does a first aid cabinet contain?

38. What is the first aid for choking? **If casualty is an adult or a child:**

   **If the casualty is an infant**:

   **If the casualty is pregnant or obese:**

39. What are the methods in giving Artificial Respiration (AR)?

40. What is the first aid for colic or abdominal spasm?

41. How can you perform obstructed airway sequence (choking) on a conscious casualty who is much taller than you?

42. How will you know if the ventilation is effective?

43. What are the priorities of first aid?

44. What is the first aid for fracture?

45. What is the purpose of "Good Samaritan" legislation for first aider?

46. How do you manage head and spinal injuries?

47. What is the first aid for deep frostbite?

48. What is the first aid for strain and sprain?

49. What is choking?

50. What are the hazards of CPR?

51. First aid for severe bleeding?

52. What will you do if you are alone and you are choked?

53. How will you know if the CPR is effective?

54. When do you administer CPR?

55. What is a splint?

56. How do you give first aid for nose bleeding?

57. What is the first aid for hypothermia?

58. How can you minimize swelling and pain?

59. What is the first aid for an open fracture bone?

60. What will you do if the casualty moves or makes noise while you are doing CPR?

61. What is cardio-pulmonary resuscitation (CPR)?

62. What is the first aid for swallowed poison?

63. When do you apply artificial respiration?

64. How do you call for medical help?

65. What will you do in case of fire?

66. What is the first aid for partially/ completely amputated limb?

    **First aid for partially amputated limb:**

    **First aid for completely amputated limb:**

67. What is the first aid for fracture?

68. What is a splint?

69. What is a joint?

What is a strain?

# MODULE
## 3
### Home Management
### Nutrition & Food Groups
### Meal Preparation
### Meal Presentation

**MODULE 3 A**

MODULE 3
A. HOME MANAGEMENT
TOTAL ALLOTTED TIME: 30 HOURS

TERMINAL OBJECTIVES OF MODULE 3 (Partial)

Upon completion of Module 3, the participant will be able to:
♦ define home and time management
♦ create a schedule of daily, weekly and monthly house chores
♦ identify various home appliances
♦ know how to use and maintain various home appliances

| TOPICS | SUB-TOPICS TOTAL TIME - 30 HRS | LEARNING SITES/TIME | | |
|---|---|---|---|---|
| | | Classroom 24 HRS. | Special Project Create a List of Chores & Schedule of Activities showing Daily, Weekly & Monthly House chores 6 hrs. | Critical Skills 8 HRS HOW TO: |
| 3.1 Home Management | 3.1.1 Definitions 3.1.2 Checklist & Schedules | 1 hr. | | a. avoid litter using storage principles b. maintain and manage a home using a systematic approach *bedroom *living room *bathrooms *kitchen c. store food in the fridge/ freezer d. clean oven/ fridge/ cupboard |
| 3.2 The Schedule of Activities | 3.2.1 Daily Routine 3.2.2 Weekly Schedule 3.2.3 Monthly Schedule 3.2.4 Assignment | 7 hrs. | | |
| 3.3 Home Appliances | 3.3.1 Uses 3.3.2 Maintenance 3.3.3 Energy Conservation 3.3.4 Individual Task Practice | 16 hrs | Practice using modern appliances | |

NOTES: *During the one-on-one assessment, the trainee must be able to verbally describe and explain the use of each of the major and small electrical appliances usually found in a home which include the vacuum cleaner, oven, stove, blender, fridge, washing machine, garborator, food processor, egg beater, clothes dryer, dishwasher, microwave oven, toaster, coffee maker, can opener. However, only the four major skills mentioned above are considered critical skills and each trainee must score 80% to pass. [In the event that the trainee scores less thant 80%, he or she must schedule another assessment until the passing mark is achieved.]
*Participants are encouraged to use the centre to hone their skills on the use of the various electrical and major appliances with the use of the INDIVIDUALIZED TASK PRACTICE SHEETS.

**MODULE 3 B**

### B. NUTRITION, BASIC FOOD PREPARATION & FOOD PRESENTATION
### TOTAL ALLOTTED TIME - 90 HOURS

TERMINAL OBJECTIVES OF MODULE 3

Upon completion of Module 3, the participant will be able to:
- understand the concept and skills in handling food and prevent contamination
- understand the concept of nutrition and food preparation
- identify the four food groups and their alternatives
- know what nutrients are and their various functions and roles in the body.
- know basic cooking terminologies
- become familiar with North American cooking
- prepare and present North American dishes
- follow recipes

### MODULE 3 OUTLINE

| TOPICS | SUB-TOPICS TOTAL TIME - 90 HRS | LEARNING SITES/TIME | | |
|---|---|---|---|---|
| | | Theoretical 30 HRS. | Lab 54 hrs | One-on-One 12 HRS |
| 4.1 The Four Food Groups | 4.1.1 Milk and Dairy Products   4.1.3 Bread & Cereal Group 4.1.2 Checklist & Schedules.   4.1.4 Fruits and Vegetables | | | |
| 4.2 Nutrients & Their Functions | 4.2.1 Basic Nutrients 4.2.2 Interlocking Patterns of Nutrients 4.2.3 Canada's Food Guide | 6 hrs. | | |
| 4.3 Basic Food Preparation/ Presentation | 4.3.1 Cooking Terminologies/ Recipes 4.3.2 Food Preparation/ Presentation *Breakfast*Lunch*Dinner/ Supper | 54 hrs (Lab) | Each group must plan, cook and serve a complete meal to a family.* | |
| 4.4 Special Project | 4.4.1 Collage Project: The Four Food Groups | | 6 hours | |
| 4.5 Food Management | 4.5.1 The Concept of Safe Food Handling 4.5.2 Prevention of Germs from Spreading 4.5.3 Food Contamination & Prevention | | 6 hours | |

*Assessment Criteria: Food Guide, Food Appeal, Before and After Preparation

TEXT: THE CAREGIVER RESOURCE MANUAL: SICES PUBLICATION
Reference: Canada Food Guide, Health Canada Publication

# CONTENTS OF MODULE 3

| 3.1 | HOME MANAGEMENT |
|-----|-----------------|

**Home Management** is the maintenance of the house which covers all domestic tasks such as the upkeep of order and cleanliness in all areas of the house, installation and replenishment of house amenities and grocery shopping list, preparation and service of food, cleaning, washing, ironing, and personal care.

### 3.1.1  THE IMPORTANCE OF CHECKLIST/SCHEDULES

**A Checklist** helps you as a caregiver maintain a fairly routine schedule without actually forgetting or ignoring the areas that require less attention.

**Housekeeping** is therefore simple provided you have systematic methods.

It is important to remember that homemaking or house chores in general are only a part of your job. Use time wisely and maintain a daily routine using the Schedule of Activities as your guide to finish tedious tasks during the early part of the morning.

### 3.1.2  NOTES/REMINDERS IN BEING ORGANIZED AND SYSTEMATIC

In addition to the above, the following suggested routine that will help you as a homemaker in being systematic and organized in your daily chores.

**Bedroom**
1. Start with the bedrooms in the morning.
2. Sheets must be changed once a week; every Monday is a good day, or any day. Meanwhile, some homes have only one change of sheets; hence, linens get washed in the morning and get put back before bedtime.
3. On any other day, the beds only need to be made.
4. In making the bed, first straighten any crinkles.
5. Then, fluff the pillows.
6. Tuck the cover or fold the cover back ¼ of the way.
7. Arrange the pillows neatly over the cover.
8. Finish by carefully covering the pillows.
9. Remove clutter and dust around.
10. It is a good idea to have a paper bag with you so little items that need sorting out could be done later on.
11. Take one last look before you leave the room. If it meets your approval, then the room is done. Move to the rest of the rooms but take a look at your checklist just be sure.

## Bathroom

1. Bathrooms are the mirrors of any home. A clean and spotless bathroom gives any home a five star approval.
2. Start cleaning the toilet bowl (inside and outside). If this is done everyday, there is no reason why it should be a major task.
3. Go over the mirror afterwards. It is really annoying to look into a dirty mirror. Toothpaste spots and finger prints are tell-tales that reveal how good a housekeeper you are.
4. Finish by polishing and shining the counter and sink. It is not enough to simply hide clutter by putting them behind the mirror and shoving them into drawers. Spend half an hour each day to major projects like cleaning shelves, drawers, etc.

## Living Room

1. The living room or family room is next in line.
2. Remove clutter, dust around.
3. Return furniture to their proper place.
4. Coffee tables must be spotless.
5. Ashtrays must be washed.

## Kitchen

1. After cleaning the living rooms, it is time to attack the kitchen.
2. Fill the sink with hot, soapy water. Soak everything that needs to be washed. If a dish washer is available, just use hot water to soak the dishes.
3. Let the dishes remain soaked while making tables, oven, fridge and counters spotless.
4. Take the head of the vacuum cleaner to groom carpets and rugs. Unless the carpet really needs vacuuming, there is no need to actually vacuum everyday, but grooming is a must.
5. Many homes are equipped with a dishwasher. Dishes need to be pre-rinsed before putting them in the dishwasher. No dishwasher can substitute for your hands in ensuring the cleanliness of the dishes. However, one very good advantage of a dishwasher is it disinfects and sanitizes dishes and utensils.
6. Now, you can go back to your dishes. It is always a good idea to rinse dishes due to some possible remnants of detergent ingredients. When using a dishwasher, simply stack the dishes and utensils in the dishwasher. Then, add detergent and run the machine. If you have enough dishes, the running of the dishwasher is saved until the end of the day.
7. Finally, you are ready for a break. The children or the elderly or the person with special needs under your charge need a mid-morning

snack, and you deserve a big cup of coffee and a sandwich or whatever snack you may prefer.

8. The whole day is now reserved for you and the person you care for. You have your peace of mind because your home is clean. It does not actually mean that your job is done, but at least for the rest of the morning you can now concentrate on providing personal care.

# 3.2 THE SCHEDULE OF ACTIVITIES

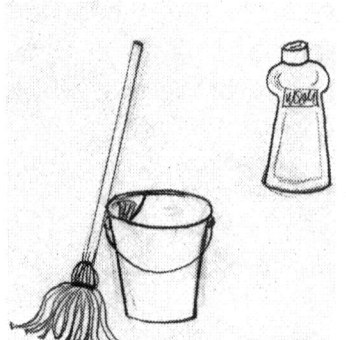

**Keeping and maintaining schedules** (e.g. daily routine, weekly and monthly schedule) is an effective tool/aid in time management. This ensures that house chores are distributed throughout the day, week, or month thereby, allowing you to keep and maintain the home in an effortless manner.

**SAMPLE:** In your journal, complete the chart using the weekly and monthly chores. In this particular example the first day of the month falls on a Thursday. For the subsequent months, it is easy to now create a schedule by ensuring that the monthly chores are filled in first. Your workshop will clarify this concept.

| Monday | Tuesday | Wednesday | Thursday | Friday |
|---|---|---|---|---|
| | | | | |
| | | | - Laundry<br>- Folding/Ironing | - Wash one wall<br>-Vacuum corridors |
| - Change bed linens<br>- Laundry | - Wash floor | - Water Plant | - Laundry<br>- Folding/Ironing | - Wash one wall<br>-Vacuum corridors |
| - Change bed linens<br>- Laundry | - Wash floor | - Water Plant | - Laundry<br>- Folding/Ironing | - Wash one wall<br>-Vacuum corridors |
| - Change bed linens<br>- Laundry | - Wash floor | - Water Plant | - Laundry<br>- Folding/Ironing | - Wash one wall<br>-Vacuum corridors |
| - Change bed linens<br>- Laundry | - Wash floor | - Water Plant | - Laundry<br>- Folding/Ironing | - Wash one wall<br>-Vacuum corridors |

Note: The daily routine is not listed in the Schedule of Activities since they are daily chores. When doing the schedule, use colored pencils to quickly identify the same chores throughout the schedule.

| *Remove Gum* | *Remove Lipstick Stains* | *Remove Red Wine Stains* |
|---|---|---|
| ❀ Put egg whites on it and leave for a few minutes on the garment or on one's hair. <br><br>*Remove Oil Stains* <br> ❀ Apply eucalyptus oil and wash with warm soapy water. <br><br>*Remove Ball-Point Pen Ink* <br> ❀ Use hairspray and rub hard with soap bar, rinse in cold water (hot water can set non-greasy stains).Do, que consua que | ❀ Apply toothpaste then wash garment as usual. <br> ❀ Or apply petroleum jelly and then wash. <br><br>*Remove Rust Stains* <br> ❀ Put some lemon juice and salt. Hang outside the sun to let it dry. <br><br>*Remove Coffee and Tea Stains* <br> ❀ Spray with hairspray and rub with soap bar. Rinse in cold water. | ❀ Wash fabric in cold water with regular detergent. <br> ❀ Wash carpets with foamy shaving cream. Rinse in cold water then vacuum dry. <br><br>*Remove Tomato-based Stains* <br> ❀ Blot it with de-natured alcohol and launder in cool water. |

## 3.2.1  DAILY ROUTINE ACTIVITIES

Go over each activity. Show that the Daily Routine Activities (the list itself) are Actual Checklists. Transfer the list of activities on a blank sheet with days of the weeks opposite them as follows.

| DAYS OF THE MONTH | | | | | | | |
|---|---|---|---|---|---|---|---|
| **AREA/ACTIVITIES** | 1 | 2 | 3 | 4 | 5 | 6 | Up to ...31 |
| **Kitchen** | | | | | | | |
| ▪ Prepare Breakfast | | | | | | | |

As you perform each activity, put a check (√) mark under the day of the month as an indicator that you performed that specific chore on that particular day. This becomes a record for each house chore that you did for the day. One advantage of this is to provide your employer with a monitor sheet at a glance.

**Kitchen**
- Prepare breakfast, lunch and supper.
- Wipe the counter top.
- Clean up or tidy up table afterwards.
- Clean the stove.
- Wash dirty dishes, and pots and pans.
- Sweep the floor.
- Load dirty dishes into the dishwasher.

**When washing**
- ❀ Always remember to dissolve soap detergents in warm or hot water before placing the dirty clothe in the washer.
- ❀ When applying, it is best to spray from the back of the fabric and not in front so that the stain won't spread deeper into the fabric.

### Bedroom
- Make the beds.
- Tidy up around the rooms.
- Dust around the area.

### Bathroom
- Wash the sink, toilet, and tub using soft cleaner.
- Clean the mirrors.
- Polish the faucets.

**Blood Stains on Clothing**
- Try applying a paste of meat tenderizing crystal and cold water and allow ½-3/4 hrs before rinsing in cold water.
- You can also apply ammonia.
- Also, foamy shaving cream used with a sponge can also help.

| **Emergency Ironing** | **Cleaning Your Iron** |
|---|---|
| 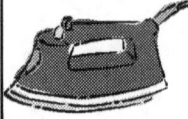 When you are in a rush and don't have time to iron, try popping the garment into the dryer with a damp towel. This will remove wrinkles in a few minutes. | Remove brown spots by rubbing with fine steel wool dipped with warm vinegar. You cal also polish it with toothpaste! Apply and let it dry. Buff with cloth. |
| **Scorched Garments** | **Non-Iron Jeans** |
| If you accidentally scorched a garment while ironing, you can sometimes salvage it by immediately soaking it in cold water overnight. | After washing, fold the jeans as you would when dry , then lay them flat on the dryer. When they come out, they will be almost as neat as if they were ironed. |

### 3.2.2  WEEKLY ROUTINE ACTIVITIES

Using the Weekly Routine Activities, locate the activities on the Schedule of Activities provided. See if you can confirm the activities listed. Ex. You must change bed linen every Monday according to the schedule.

1. Laundry twice a week.
   - Separate the whites from the colored clothes.
   - Check the machine and hand washable.
   - Separate the hand washable.
   - Separate the ones that are to be dry cleaned.
2. Fold clothes, towels, linen etc. when done and put them in their proper places.
3. Change bed linen once a week.
4. Water plants.

5. Vacuum all over, twice in traffic areas.
6. General dusting (i.e. coffee table, end tables, etc.).
7. Wash kitchen floor and some uncarpeted areas.
8. Wash walls.

### 3.2.3  MONTHLY ROUTINE ACTIVITIES

Using the Monthly Routine Activities, locate the activities on the Schedule of Activities provided below, see if you can confirm the activities listed. Ex: You must clean the oven on the third Tuesday of each month. Finish putting the rest of the activities on the Schedule of Activities sheet.

1. Wash the fridge.
2. Clean the cupboards.
3. Clean the oven; check if it's self-cleaning.
4. Vacuum the sofa, chesterfield, or chairs.
5. Vacuum the drapes.
6. Clean the windows (inside part).
7. Dust pictures and paintings.
8. Clean the kitchen drawers.
9. Tidy up the children's drawers.

### 3.2.4  WORKSHOP: CREATE  YOUR OWN SCHEDULE OF HOUSE CHORES

*Note: Using your scheduling skills you should be able to do a schedule of personal care when you get to those modules.*

## 3.3　HOME APPLIANCES (USES, MAINTENANCE, AND ENERGY CONSERVATION)

In this modern age, majority of the homes are equipped with commonly used home appliances which when used properly, makes life more enjoyable and convenient. The uses and maintenance of these appliances must be learned in order to avoid unnecessary accidents, thereby maintaining safety in the home. As many of the appliances are electric, conservation of energy must also be observed. Unnecessary use of power is not only a waste of money but a very bad habit to acquire. Especially with children, you model what you expect.

### 3.3.1 CARING FOR AND MAINTENANCE OF KITCHEN APPLIANCES (HINTS)

Following are some pointers in maintaining and removing stains in some kitchen appliances:

***Shiny Appliances***
- To keep appliances shiny, wipe them with a cloth or sponge wrung out in lukewarm soapy water. Rinse and wipe dry with a soft cloth or remove water pots.

***Chrome-trimmed Appliances***
- Wipe any chrome-trimmed appliances such as toaster with a soft cloth moistened in rubbing alcohol to keep it shining always.

***Removing Rust from Kitchen Chrome***
- To remove rust from kitchen chrome, wrap an aluminum foil around your finger, shiny side out, and rub the rust until it disappears. Then wipe the surface with a damp cloth and polish with a dry cloth.

***Removing Dust Underneath Appliances***
- Use a snow brush (the long handle type used to brush and scrape snow from the car's windshield) to whisk dirt from under and behind kitchen appliances such as fridge and freezers that are not on casters. Be sure to unplug any of the appliances before cleaning it or around it.

***Removing Spills/Grease***

    a. **Stovetop**
- Always wipe spills and splattered grease on the stovetop while cooking surfaces are still warm. Use a sponge or cloth wrung in soapy water then rinse.
- The coils or cooking surfaces on top of the stove do not require any cleaning because the spill are usually burned off.

    b.   **Oven**
- Prevent spill built up by washing and wiping out inside and outside the oven after its use. Otherwise the grease will harden and burn each time you turn the oven.

**c. Oven Racks and Pots and Pans**
- A solution of ammonia and hot water is a good cleaning solution for oven racks and greasy pots and pans. Be sure to rinse well.
- While pots, pans, frying pans, roasting ovens are still hot after cooking; scrape as much as the foodstuff from each, pour dishwasher detergent, fill it with water, and let it soak. This procedure will soften all burnt food hence cleaning becomes no chore at all.

**d. Refrigerator Top**
- Sticky, greasy top part of a refrigerator can be cleansed with a solution of 1 part ammonia to 10 parts water. Once the solution has broken down the grease, wipe with a soft cloth wrung from a soapy water, and rinse.

**e. Coffee Maker**
- Thoroughly clean the coffee maker once a month with equal parts of water and vinegar. Rinse by running clear water through the cycle.

**f. Food Blender or Food Processor**
- To clean a food blender or a food processor, partly fill it with water and a small amount of manual dishwashing detergent. Cover and run the blender for a few seconds. Rinse and dry.

**g. Porcelain Sinks**
- For porcelain sinks, remove stains by filling it with water and small amount of chlorine bleach. Let stand for an hour. Rinse and wipe dry.
- For stubborn stains at the bottom, line it with three layers of paper towels. Pour and saturate the towels with concentrated bleach. Let it stand overnight.
- The above procedure is not recommended for cracked or chipped porcelain surface because the bleach can penetrate the iron base that will cause rusting.

**h. Countertops, etc.**
- For counter tops, sinks, cutting board, butcher blocks, kitchen tables and cupboards, baking soda will clean and deodorize the appliances.
- For stain marks, make a baking soda paste by dripping a small amount of water on to a generous amount of baking soda. Coat and rub the surface. Wipe clean, rinse, and dry.

## 3.3.2 ELECTRICAL APPLIANCES

Following are various commonly used electrical appliances at home and their specific purposes/uses, parts and functions, and proper usage. It is always important to note that when plugging electrical appliances to power supply, be sure to have dry hands and to stand on dry ground/area to prevent any electric shock.

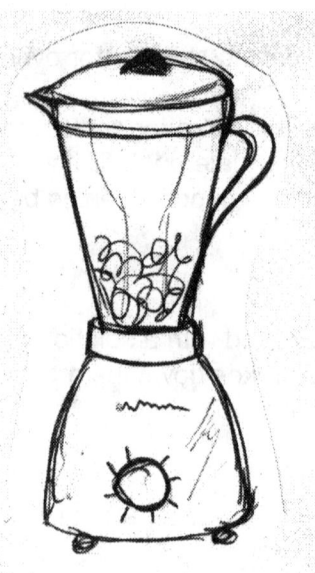

### a.    Blender/Osterizer

An electrical appliance/ device used to mix thoroughly two or more ingredients until it smoothens.

### Parts and their Function:

1.    Specification table - where the voltage, watts, and cycle of the equipment is specified.
2.    Electrical plug/cord - to connect/disconnect from power supply.
3.    Quadripods - supports the whole device.
4.    Motor - makes possible the mixing of all the ingredients.
5.    Cover/ lid - serves as protection to prevent contamination and spillage.
6.    Switch selector - determines the mixing mode and types of ingredients to be mixed.
7.  Handle - for easy handling/ transport of the device.
8.  Blade - responsible for mixing the ingredients.

### Proper Use of Blender:

1. Rinse the appliance/ device thoroughly.
2. Check if the machine voltage corresponds with the main voltage in your home.
3. Prepare the ingredients to be mixed.
4. Fill the jug with the ingredients and the desired amount of water.
5. Cover it and position to the motor.
6. Press the selector switches. Wait until the ingredients/mixture smoothens.

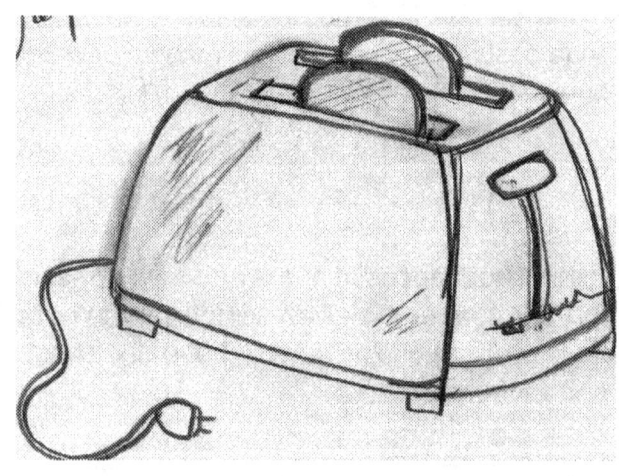

### b.    Bread Toaster

An appliance or device solely used for toasting sliced bread only. To keep the toast

hot, toasting of bread should only be done if the person to be served is about to eat.

### Parts and their Function:

1.    Specification table - where the voltage, watts, and cycle of the equipment specified.
2. Electrical plug/ cord - to connect/ disconnect from power supply.
3. Quadripods - supports the whole device.
4. Handle - for easy handling/ transport of the device.

5. Body - supports the internal parts of the device.
6. Bread grills - the heated part where toasting actually takes place.
7. Lever - lowers the sliced bread, to bread grills, and release toast automatically.
8. Toast regulator - for selecting the desired color of toasted bread.

**Proper Use of Bread Toaster:**
1. Determine the voltage of the toaster and look for compatible socket and plug it with dry hands.
2. Place the sliced bread into bread grills.
3. Lower the bread by putting down the lever. Set the indicator for desired color of the toast. Wait for the lever to go up and release the bread.
4. To avoid electric shock, unplug the power source before removing bread from toaster by using fork. Remember that fork is made of metal which is a conductor of electricity.
5. After using, unplug the toaster from the power supply with a dry hand. Let it cool down before turning it upside down to remove breadcrumbs. Open the base of the toaster by pressing the lock. Remove the breadcrumbs that stick to it by brushing. Close the base lock and set the toaster aside.

c. **Coffee Maker**
An appliance or device used for making coffee in the shortest time possible.

**Parts and their Functions:**
1. Specification table - where the voltage, watts, and cycle of the equipment specified.
2. Electrical plug/ cord - to connect/disconnect from power supply.
3. Quadripods - supports the whole device
4. Tank/ Decanter with water level - container for water (cold) to be processed.
5. Measuring scoop - used to measure coffee.
6. Carafe or jug - container for brewed coffee.
7. Cover/ lid - to protect/ cover the water from spilling during the operation.
8. Hot plate - maintains the temperature of the brewed coffee.
9. Filter cone/ Brewing funnel - receptacle for filter with ground coffee.
10. On/Off switch - for starting/ stopping the motor.

**Proper Use of Coffee Maker:**
1. Remove the brewing funnel. Place coffee (ground) into the filter.
2. Make sure the filter and carafe are in the proper position.
3. Fill the decanter/ water tank with water to desired capacity as marked on the side of the decanter, (1 cup = 5 oz). (To brew 10 cups of coffee, fill the decanter to the bottom of the silver band).
4. Lift the water tank cover and pour the water into the tank. Cover then

switch on to desired power supply.

5. Wash the decanter, lid, carafe, and brewing funnel in a mixture of mild detergent and water. Rinse each thoroughly.
6. If you have a clock model, set the clock. The digital clock model must be set first before the coffee maker will operate.
7. Slide the brewing funnel into the right place.
8. When the brewing cycle is finished, turn your coffee maker off. Discard the water in the decanter. Rinse the decanter and brewing funnel.

### 3-7

### d. Electric Skillet

An appliance or device used for cooking pot roast, stir-frying and broiling, etc. It is stick/non- stick pan with cover, handle, temperature regulator and quadripods.

### Parts and their Functions:

Specification table - where the voltage, watts and cycle of the equipment is specified.

Electrical plug/ cord - to connect/ disconnect from power supply.

### Proper Use of an Electric Skillet:

1. Plug it to appropriate power supply and set the thermostat to desired temperature.
2. Inspect the meat once in a while and turn it from the side to cook it evenly.
3. When nearly done switch it off. Do not remove the cover. Let the remaining heat cook the meat.
4. After cooking, remove the food from the pan and transfer it to another container. Cover it.
5. Allow it to cool down. Then clean it with water and detergent. Scrub the pan, if necessary.
6. Rinse it well. Set aside with topside down to dry it.
7. Before using the skillet, determine the voltage and identify a socket compatible to the voltage.
8. With a dry hand while stepping on a dry surface, plug it to power supply.
9. Disconnect the skillet from power supply when cooking is nearly done.

### 3-8

### e. Refrigerator (Fridge)

An appliance or device used for preserving, storing, cooling, freezing foods, drinks and medicines to keep them from spoiling. It uses electric power and freon gas to cool the internal parts of the fridge.

**Parts and their Functions:**
1. Specification table - where the voltage, watts and cycle of the equipment is specified.
2. Electrical plug/ cord - to connect/ disconnect from power supply.
3. Motor- located at the back lower portion - makes possible the cooling of the fridge.
4. Condenser coils - located at the back, it holds the freon that cools the whole system.
5. Thermostat - regulates temperature inside the fridge.
6. Freezer - the coldest part, used for storing meat, fish, poultry, ice cream, and salads.
7. Chiller - storage compartment under freezer for the cold cuts like ham, bacon, sausages, etc.
8. Crisper - storage compartment for vegetables.
9. Racks/ grill - storage for drinks and left over foods.
10. Door with gasket - protects the food from contamination and seals the internal coolness of the fridge.
11. Egg rack - holds the eggs.
12. Cheese rack - storage compartment for cheese or butter.
13. Medicine rack - storage area for medicines.
14. Portable bins - storage of bottle drinks.
15. Bulb - for internal illumination.

**Proper Use of the Fridge:**
1. Store foods, food containers, drinks, and medicines in their proper places.
2. Determine the voltage of the equipment and look for compatible socket. Plug to proper supply with a dry hand.
3. Turn the thermostat to the required temperature then close the door firmly.
4. Prior to defrosting, turn the thermostat to off or defrost position for at least overnight.
5. The following morning, unplug and remove all the contents of the fridge. Set it aside.
6. Clean the food compartments with soft detergents and rinse with water. Wipe with dry cloth. Restore the food to appropriate compartments and dispose the foods that are nearly spoiled, dried or rotten. Place a charcoal cup in a hidden corner inside the fridge to absorb odors. With a dry hand, plug it to the power supply and turn the thermostat to required temperature.
7. Don't pile soft fruits in storage.
8. Don't store fruits in ward placer unless you want to speed ripening.
9. Store potatoes, onions, beets, carrots, and other root vegetables in a cool, dry, well-ventilated area. Keep other vegetables in crisper of refrigerator.

## f. Microwave Oven

**3-9**

An electrical appliance or device used for cooking, pre-heating, defrosting frozen meat in the shortest possible time. It consumes so much electricity that is converted by motor into microheat waves that makes cooking of foods as fast as possible.

### Parts and their Functions:
1. Specification table - where the voltage, watts, and cycle of the equipment is specified.
2. Electrical plug/ cord - to connect/ disconnect from power supply.
3. High visible door- to see the food inside when cooking /defrosting
4. Selector switches:
   a. defrost
   b. cook
   c. timer
   d. bell - rings as timer zero in to remind that cooking pre-heating or defrosting is done.
5. Door button - for door opening
6. Rollers - responsible for turning the removable glass tray.
7. Hatches - used to secure the content of the oven.
8. Removable glass tray - serves as food receptacle when cooking
9. Stirrer - outlet for heatwave.

### Proper Use of Microwave:
1. From the specification table, determine the voltage of the microwave oven and look for compatible socket to avoid short circuit.
2. When pre-heating or cooling, the pointer should be on the proper position, and defrost position, if defrosting.
3. Open the door by pushing the door button.
4. Place the food for pre-heating/ cooking or defrosting at the center of the glass tray then close the door firmly by pushing manually.
5. With a dry hand, plug it to the electric power supply.
6. Position the timer. Switch to required time and close the door.
7. As the timer zero-in, the bell will ring to remind that cooking is done. Disconnect from power supply.

## g. Rice Cooker

An electrical appliance or device used for cooking rice, boiling dish and sterilizing nursing bottles. It comes in different sizes and capacity.

### Parts and their Function:
1. Specification table - where the voltage, watts and cycle of the equipment is specified.
2. Electrical plug/ cord - to connect/disconnect from power supply.

3. Hot plate - the heated part that actually cooks rice on the receptacle.
4. Switch on/off - for cooking and warming of rice.
5. Receptacle - holds the cereal and water for cooking.
6. Handle - for easy lifting and transport of the device.
7. Cover - protects the food from contamination.

**Proper Use of the Rice Cooker:**
1. Determine the voltage of rice cooker and look for compatible socket to avoid short circuit. Put into the receptacle the rice grains for washing. Then add water in equal ratio (1 cup of water : 1 cup of grains).
2. Wipe with dry cloth the base of receptacle to prevent water from dripping on the hot plate which results to cracking sounds. Put the cover. To avoid electric shock, plug to power supply with a dry hand. Press down the cook switch and transfer to warm position.
3. With a dry hand, disconnect it from the power source. The remaining heat will keep the rice warm. If the all cooked rice is consumed, wash the receptacle with water and detergents. Set the receptacle aside, up side down to dry it.
4. If there are still some rice, place the receptacle back on the rice cooker. Wash the cover and remove spills then put the cover back. To reheat rice, plug it to the power supply by pressing switch to cook position. No need to add water.

**h. Oven Toaster**

An electrical appliance or device used for roasting, cooking, pre-heating, and toasting.

**Parts and their Function:**
1. Specification table - where the voltage, watts and cycle of the equipment is specified.
2. Electrical plug/ cord - to connect/ disconnect from power supply.
3. Quadripods - supports the whole device.
4. Baking rack - supports the oven tray while cooking.
5. Heating elements/ quartz heater - makes cooking possible.
6. See-through oven window - to see if food is done.
7. Door handle - for easy opening and closing of door.
8. Timer - will remind you if cooking is done.

**Proper Use of Oven Toaster:**
1. Plug in power cord directly into a tight filling wall outlet. See that full length of plug pins are properly inserted.
2. Open the oven door and place food on baking rack. Close the oven door.
3. Turn on the timer clockwise, to turn the switch on. Set it at proper cooking time. When setting time for 5 minutes or less, first turn the timer beyond 6 minutes and then return to desired setting.

**After Care of Oven Toaster:**
1. Always unplug power cord and allow oven toaster to cook before cleaning.
2. Periodically open the crumb tray and remove breadcrumbs from the bottom of oven toaster.
3. Clean exterior surfaces with soft damp cloth. Do not use abrasive cleaners or metal scourging pads.
4. Clean interior surface with damp soft cloth dip in warm water.
5. Wash oven tray in warm water and wipe with soft dry cloth.

**i. Vacuum Cleaner**

An appliance or device that uses a motor that picks up dust and other tiny solid particles in carpet.

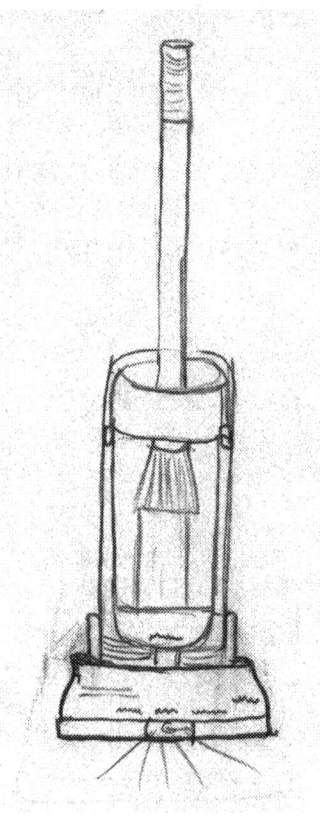

**Parts and their Function:**
1. Specification table - where the voltage, watts, and cycle of the equipment is specified.
2. Electrical plug/ cord - to connect/ disconnect from power supply.
3. Motor - makes possible the sucking of dust, dirt, and liquid waste.
4. Switch on/ off - for starting and stopping the operation.
5. Filter - for circulation of air inside the bucket
6. Waste tank/ bucket - container for dirt or liquid waste.
7. Extension tubes - for reaching far areas.
8. Castors - consists of 4 rollers for support and mobility.
9. Flexible hose - connects from inlet to extension tubes.
10. Nozzles - the portion that actually touches the surface like ceiling, walls, floors and corners.
11. Inlet hole - the opening into the bucket and used when draining dirt or fluid waste.
12. Latches - used to secure the content of the bucket/ waste tank.

**Proper Use of Vacuum Cleaner:**
1. See to it that the area to be vacuumed/ cleaned is clear of any materials you do not wish to be sucked into the vacuum. Determine the voltage of the machine and look for the compatible socket to avoid short circuit.
2. Start the vacuum cleaner by pressing the ON switch (OFF switch to stop it). Position the vacuum's body and start vacuuming the place by aiming the extension tubes for easy sucking of dirt.

3. If done, turn off the power switch and disconnect the plug from power supply. Disconnect from the bucket/waste tank all the parts of the vacuum cleaner, including its motor. Empty the bucket by disposing the contents to the garbage can. Set aside vacuum for future use.

### j. Washing Machine
An electrical appliance or device used for washing, disinfecting, rinsing and drying clothes and fabrics

### Parts and their Function:
1. Specification table - where the voltage, watts, and cycle of the equipment is specified.
2. Electrical plug/ cord - to connect/ disconnect from power supply.
3. Cover/ lid - prevents water from spilling and keeps clothes from flying during drying.
4. Surgilator- makes possible the rotation of laundry in the tub.
5. Tub - dispenser for clothes to be washed.
6. Control panel
   a. Load size selector - determines the amount of clothes to be washed
   b. Temperature selector - determines the temperature of water to be used.
   c. Timer - regulates the time requirement during washing, rinsing, and drying.
7. Drainage hose - exit of water and detergent during rinsing.
8. Water supply hose - supplies water from tap to the tub.
9. Ground wire - used to prevent electric shock.
10. Motor - responsible for washing, rinsing, and drying.
11. Quadripods - holds the whole device.

### Proper Use of Washing Machine:
1. Sort the clothes first:

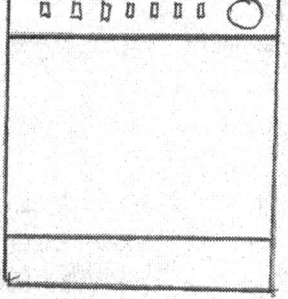

   a. Separate the whites and the colored clothes.
   b. Separate the machine washables from hand washables.
   c. Button the unbutton.
   d. Zip the unzip.
   e. Turn the pockets into wrong side position.
   f. Separate the light colors from the heavy dark color.
2. Fill the tub with water up to ¾ and add detergent depending upon the load size.
3. Put the laundry into the tub.
4. Close the lid and position the selector switches

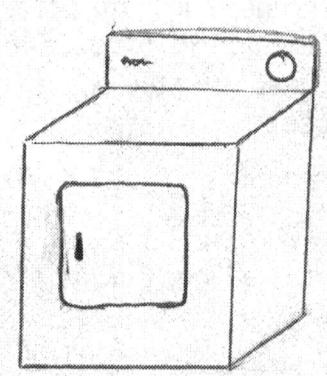

depending upon washing requirement.

5.    With a dry hand, plug it to power supply and pull the timer switch to start.

6.    If done, push down the timer switch before unplugging from the power source. Open the lid. Retrieve the clothes, turn to wrong side, and hang.

## k.  Dishwashing Machine

An electrical appliance or device used for cleaning, disinfecting, rinsing, and drying dishes like plates, cups, glasses, saucers, and pot and pans. It has a component that heats water and detergent being sprayed with force to dishes.

### Parts and their Functions:

1.                                 **3-13**

2. Specification table - where the voltage, watts, and cycle of the equipment is specified.
3. Electrical plug/ cord - to connect/ disconnect from power supply.
4. Water supply hose - for water supply inside the washer dish.
5. Draining hose - for draining detergent and used water after rinsing.
6. Door with gasket - seals the detergent and hot water during washing and rinsing process.
7. Selector switches - determines the cleaning mode and types of dishes to be cleaned.
8. Top rack - dispenser for glasses and cups and saucers.
9. Bottom rack - dispenser for plates, and pots and pans.
10. Side rack - dispenser for silverwares, ladles, and cutleries.
11. Iron coil - located at the base inside, which makes possible the heating of water during the cleaning process.
12. Motor - makes possible the processes of cleaning, disinfecting, and rinsing.
13. Drainage holes - exit of remaining food particles, detergent, and hot water inside the washer dish.
14. Soap dispenser - holds the soap (bar or powder only) for washing the dishes.

### Proper Use of Dishwashing Machine:

1.    Get the soiled dishes ready by scraping large food particles on the surface. Open dishwasher's door by pressing the lock. Position the glasses upside down on the top rack, occupying two prongs each and leave one prong in between to avoid breaking of glasses.

2. Arrange the saucers and cups on the left side of top rack. Keep their distance from each other to avoid breakage. Arrange the plates and pots and pans facing downward on the bottom rack.
3. Place the silverwares, ladles, and cutleries on the side rack at the inner portion of the door. Put some detergent on the soap dispenser and close the door gently. With a dry hand, plug it and position the selector switches to start.

## I. Gas Range

An electrical appliance or device used for cooking, baking that sues liquified petroleum gas or fuel. It has gas burners and an electrical hot plate that uses electric power.

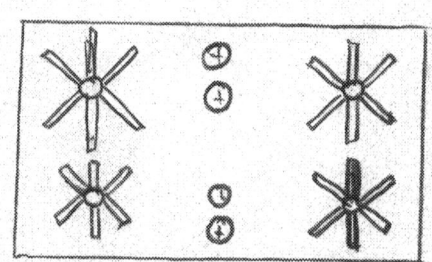

**Parts and their Functions:**
1. Specification table - where the voltage, watts, and cycle of the equipment is specified.
2. Electrical plug/ cord - to connect/ disconnect from power supply.
3. Cover- to keep the burners and the hot plate from sight and for protection also.
4. Burners - for equal distribution of flame/ heat.
5. Flame switches - regulates the heat on burners and ovens.
6. Tripods - holds the cooking utensils over the burners.
7. Hose and gas regulators - regulates the release of the gas from the cylinder.
8. Oven - used for baking, roasting, and pre-heating pies.
9. Racks - holds the baking pans, cookie sheets, and pan for pre-heating.
10. Rotisserie - holds the meats for roasting.
11. Grill - dispenser for rotisserie.

**Proper Use of Electric/Gas Range:**
1. After preparing the food to be cooked, select the burner that fits the cooking utensils. (Big burners for big pans while small burners for small pans for economic fuel consumption).
2. To prevent gas leaks, make sure that all flame regulators are closed before turning on the gas regulator.

**Oven Spills**
- When spills occur, sprinkle with table salt. When the oven cools, wipe off the salt which has already absorbed the drippings.

**Sparkling Oven Tops**
- Use rubbing alcohol for beautiful, shiny oven tops.

**Cleaning Matte-covered Counters**
- Apply club soda, rinse with warm water, dry. Simply wipe with wet clean and do not use abrasive cleaners.

**Instant Kitchen Deodorizer**
- In a pan of boiling water, sprinkle cinnamon.

**Easily Pick-up Broken Glass**
- Use a slice of fresh bread to pick up tiny pieces of broken glass.

**Easily Clean Spilled Egg**
- If you accidentally dropped egg on the kitchen floor, sprinkle some salt to absorb the egg and allow you to mop it with a cloth or paper towel.

4. In cooking dishes with vegetables, switch off the burner's flame and let the remaining heat cook the vegetables. Let the dish cool down on the burner before cleaning.
5. After closing the gas regulator and flame switches, clean the stovetop by wiping spills with damp cloth.
6. Before using the oven, check if it is clean.
7. Pre-heat the oven while preparing something to be baked/ roasted.
8. Inspect the thermostat and check for the desired temperature.
9. If the cookie sheets or baking pans are ready, open the oven door and place them properly on the rack. Close the door as soon as possible to prevent heat release. Observe cooking time of set timer, if it has any.
10. Inspect the food through visible door. If necessary, interchange cookie sheets using potholders, or check the food if it is done.

### Gelatin Tip

❀ Always soften gelatin first in cold water and dissolve it in hot water. If you let the water boil, the gelatin could lose it's gelatin properties.

### When baking bananas for dessert

❀ Dip the bananas in juice first to lessen chances of burning them up when baking.

### Cutting marshmallows

❀ Simply put some flour on scissors and cut.

### Storing Coffee Beans

❀ Coffee beans stay fresh longer when kept in the freezer of your fridge.

Sugar on Cold Drinks

❀ Always dissolve sugar in a little hot water to prevent it from sinking to the bottom of cold drinks.

### Crisping Wilted Lettuce

❀ Add a few drops of lemon juice or cider vinegar to a bowl of ice cold water. Add the wilted lettuce and let is stand for 1 hour.

### Non-Sticky Rice

❀ Add lemon juice to boiling rice to prevent grains from sticking together.

Rescuing Burnt Rice

❀ Place a slice of brad on top of the slightly burned rice to absorb its burnt taste.

### Moist Meatballs

❀ Place a small ice-cube chip at the center of each meatball to prevent the meatball from drying while being cooked.

### Sausages

❀ Boil for 5 to 10 minutes and roll in flour before frying or broiling to remove excess fats and keep prevent sausage shrinkage.

### When Cooking Roasts

❀ To ensure moistness of roast, add salt when the roast is nearly cooked. Otherwise, the salt will draw all the juices out from the roast.

❀ You can also place some celery sticks under the roast which will make the cleaning of pan easier

❀ If you will cook a tough roast, place a banana or slices of pineapple to tenderize the meat.

# 3.4 Basic Food Preparation And Presentation

## 3.4.1 SAFETY PRECAUTIONS AND PRACTICES TO BE OBSERVED IN THE KITCHEN

The kitchen can be the most dangerous place in the home. Real kitchen safety depends upon good work habits. Slips/falls on the floors cause the greatest number of accidents in the homes. Scalds and burns are second. The following rules will help avoid accidents:

1.  **Plan.** Plan your work so that there is no last minute dashing around. Hurrying can cause slipping and serious injury.
2.  **Appropriate attire, tools, job.** Use the proper attire. Note the proper use of tools for the appropriate job/ task.
3.  **No hand jewelry.** Remove all hand jewelry when working in the kitchen.
4.  **Wash hands.** Wash your hands before doing any work.
5.  **Use potholders.** Use potholders whenever handling hot utensils.
6.  **Orderliness/Cleanliness.** Keep orderliness and cleanliness in the kitchen. Put things in their proper places. Any object left out of place may be dangerous.
7.  **Non-skid mats.** Place nonskid, sponge rubber mats by the sink and range.
8.  **Gas Ranges.** If at all possible, have ranges out of reach of a window to prevent curtains from catching fire. Otherwise, select short curtains.
9.  **Pots and pans handles**. Turn the handles of pots and pans away from the edges of the stove.
10. **Loose pan handles.** Repair or discard pans with loose handle.
11. **Wrong use of Apron.** Avoid using the corner of your apron instead of potholders because if a hot pan is held, it can easily be dropped.
12. **Wipe spills.** Wipe off spills immediately. Slipping can cause serious injury.
13. **Short circuits.** Inspect the cords of all kitchen appliances used for frying. Short circuits can cause house fire.
14. **Cords.** Place all cords out of children's reach; place them where children cannot be tripped over. Teach your children not to tamper with electrical equipment, floor plugs, and sockets. Never use a wet cord.
15. **Knives.** Avoid placing knives in a sink of soapy water.
16. **Wall can opener / electric can opener.** Both a can opener and a can cover can be dangerous. It is a good idea to invest in a wall can opener or an electric can opener because with these, no jagged edges are left on the can opener.
17. **No toys.** Be sure no toys are left in the floor to stumble over.
18. **Slotted Racks for Knives.** Knives placed together in a drawer are dangerous. The edges are also dulled and nicked. The best place to store knives is in slotted racks.
19. **Broken glasses.** Clean up broken glass immediately but carefully. The smallest pieces can be picked up with a damp piece of paper.
20. **Fires.** Learn how to handle fires – throw salt in a grease fire if you do not have a fire extinguisher.

## 3.4.2 PROPER HAND-WASHING PROCEDURE

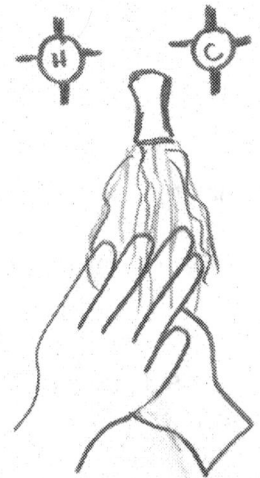

### *Steps:*

1. Gather the needed materials for hand washing. The germicidal soap with nailbrush for the caregiver and the hand towel.
2. Open the faucet; regulate the water temperature. Wet hands. Apply soap; form a lather by rubbing palms together. Pay attention in between fingers wherein most bacteria stay.
3. Use circular motion in cleaning hands up to 2 to 3 inches below the wrist.
4. Brush the nails. Rinse thoroughly.
5. Let the water drip off your hands by raising it up with palms facing the chest.
6. Pat and dry from the cleanest to the dirtiest.
7. Discard the hand towel to the laundry basket.

## 3.4.3 COOKING TERMINOLOGIES

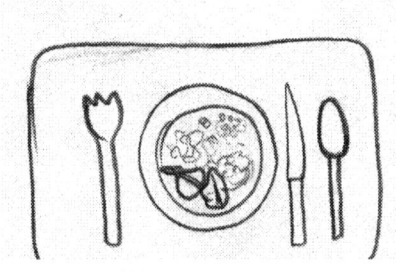

**Bake** : To cook food in the oven (cake, meat, cookies, etc)

**Boil** : To cook by immersing the food in a pan of liquid which must be kept boiling gently at all times.

**Braise** : A combination of stewing and roasting. Meat is placed on a bed of vegetables with little liquid surrounding it. In a covered vessel, cook it slowly in the oven.

**Broil** : To cook directly under heating unit in range, or over hot coals.

**Casserole** : A type of cooking food together (meat, vegetables, etc.) in a covered dish in the oven.

| | |
|---|---|
| **Chop** | : To cut food into pieces. |
| **Cube** | : To dice or cut food into small equal-sized pieces (1/4 to ½ inch squares). |
| **Deep Fried** | : To cook by immersing the food in a deep pan full of oil.. |
| **Dot** | : To drop bits of butter or cheese here and there over food. |
| **Garnish** | : To decorate food before serving. |
| **Grate** | : To rub against a grater to produce small pieces. |
| **Grill** | : To cook quickly under a red hot grill. This is used for small tender pieces of meat, fish, etc. |
| **Grease** | : To spread the bottom and sides of pan with shortening to stop food from sticking to it. |
| **Fry** | : To cook in a frying in very little oil. |
| **Marinade** | : To soak meat, or fish in a concoction of herbs, wines spices, etc. for sometime before being cooked to improve their flavour. |
| **Melt** | : To heat solids into the liquid state. |
| **Mince** | : To chop or cut into tiny pieces, the size of rice. |
| **Pan Fry** | : To cook in small amount of fat or oil in a skillet. (See Fry also). |
| **Pare** | : To cut off outside skin, as from an apple or potato. |
| **Peel** | : To pull off outer skin, as from an orange or banana. |
| **Poach** | : To cook (usually eggs or fish) gently in shallow water just below boiling point. |
| **Pressure Cooking** | : Cooking under high pressure, in a tightly covered pan. |
| **Roast** | : To cook in a hot oven or an open fire. |
| **Season** | : To add salt, pepper, spices, or herbs to food to give it more flavour. |
| **Shred** | : To cut into very thin strips |
| **Sift** | : To pass through to sieve or sifter to remove lumps in flour, sugar etc. |
| **Simmer** | : To cook just below boiling point so that the liquid bubbles gently at the sides of the pan. |
| **Slice** | : To cut into thin broad pieces. |
| **Steam** | : To cook either in a steamer over a pan of boiling water. |
| **Stew** | : To cook slowly until the food is tender. It is done when there is just enough liquid to cover the food. This liquid should be rich and is served with the food. Stew maybe cooked in a covered saucepan, casserole on a hot plate, or in the oven, but always at a low temperature. |
| **Toss** | : To mix lightly, usually salads. |

## 3.4.4  FOOD PREPARATION AND PRESENTATION

## SCIENTIFIC PRINCIPLES OF COOKING

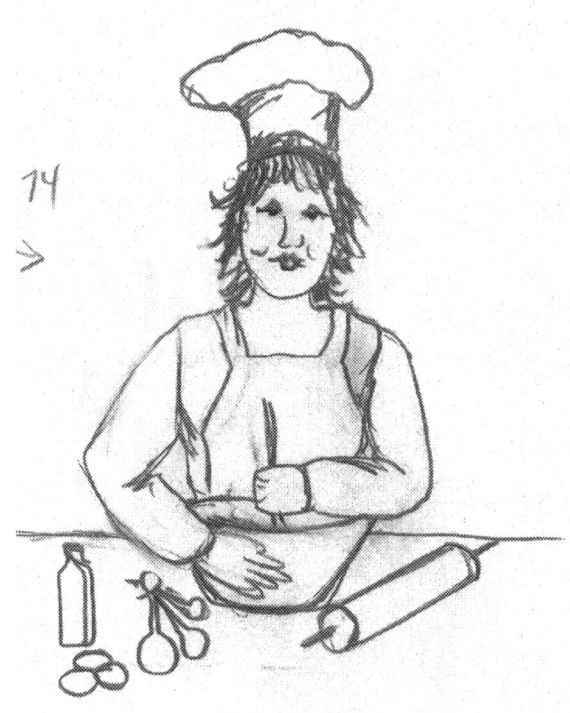

Food is cooked to bring about desirable results namely:

➤ To kill harmful microorganisms and parasites,

➤ To destroy anti-digestive factors specially beans, peas, and cereals, to preserve food,

➤ To soften tissues, bones cellulose (texture changes),

➤ To bring about color and flavor changes,

➤ To develop a more palatable product, and

➤ To have variety in food preparation.

## EGG COOKERY

Eggs vary widely in freshness, size and quality. Gauging these said factors and understanding their effects are the keys to successful egg cookery. Of the three variables, freshness is the hardest one to assess.

### *Gauging Freshness of Eggs*

▪ A fresh egg will contain a well-centered yolk, surrounded by a viscous white substance. More than five-sixths of the egg white is water; the remainder is virtually pure protein, in the form of the transparent substances known as albumin. The egg yolk contains more protein than the white, as well as vitamins, minerals, and a plenty supply of fat.

▪ Class A eggs must have rough, clean, undamaged shells.

▪ Another way of roughly gauging the freshness of an egg is to shake it gently close to your ear. There will be no audible movement in a really fresh egg, but you will hear the contents of an older egg shifting inside the shell.

### *Storing Eggs*

▪ Eggs, however fresh, must be stored correctly, in a cool place at a constant temperature – ideally between 7° and 13° Centigrade (45 ° and 55 ° F) – or in the least cold part of the refrigerator. The pores in their shells make eggs vulnerable to invasion of airborne bacteria and odors. Keep eggs away from strong-smelling foods.

### Techniques/Ways of Cooking Eggs

- The following are techniques/ways of cooking eggs namely: boiled, poached, scrambled, sunny side-up, cloudy, over-easy, omelet, and French toast.
- Whether fried, boiled, poached or baked, whole eggs (those what are not eaten before cooking), share a need for gentle heat. Low temperature keeps the whites from being rubbery and risk of firming up the yolks.
- The firm, well-centered yolks and cohesive whites of fresh eggs are particularly advantageous for poaching or frying. It is best to use slightly older eggs when boiling for shelling. The contents of new laid eggs cling so closely to the shell membrane that the eggs are difficult to peel. Eggs that are two to three weeks old, while no less nutritious than fresher eggs, are best used where appearances is not a factor for baking or in sauces.

### Utensils

- Non-stick frying pan, apron, fork, spatula, plate, Stove, pot holder,  c o v e r, table

### Ingredients

- Milk, bread, salt, milk, oil, water, pepper, sugar

### HOW TO COOK EGGS

It is best to know how to cook eggs properly. The important thing to remember is to cook eggs in very little oil (if required) or no oil at all.

**1. Boiled**

a.	Gather all needed tools and materials.

b.	Arrange the eggs loosely in a saucepan.

c.	Cover them generously with water and place the pan over a medium heat. Time the eggs from the moment the bubbles begin to rise from the bottom of the pan. Adjust the heat to maintain a bare simmer.

d.	When the eggs have cooked from the time required, remove them from the pan and immediately plunge them into cold water to stop further cooking. Cook for 4 minutes if you want it soft-boiled. Cook for 6 minutes if you want it hard-boiled.

**2. Cloudy**

a.	Gather all needed tools and materials.

b.	Set the stove in low Temperature.

c.	Grease the pan with small amount of oil only.

d.	When hot, break one egg into the pan, then add salt (optional).

e.	Put small amount of water, then add salt.

f. Cover.

g. When white covering appears on the yolk, remove from pan and the cooking is done.

h. Turn off the stove.

## 3. French Toast

a. Gather the needed tools and materials, heat the pan.

b. Break 2 eggs in a bowl, add milk then stir.

c. Dip the sliced bread quickly on both sides.

d. Reduce heat to medium setting.

e. Fry bread until golden brown, then turn over.

f. When cooked, butter bread and serve while still hot with syrup.

g. Turn off the stove.

## 4. Omelet

a. Gather all needed tools and materials.

b. Break egg into a bowl and beat until frothy.

c. Set the stove in low Temperature (omelets, on the other hand, are normally cooked over high heat, to create firm outer casings with soft interior).

d. Grease the pan.

e. Pour the beaten egg in the pan, stir while adding milk.

f. When firm, add fillings (diced onions, ham, green pepper, etc) and fold three times or turn it over to finish cooking. Serve.

h. Turn off the gas regulator.

## 5. Over-Easy

a. Same as in Sunny side-up until done.

b. Turn it over to one side for at least 10 seconds.

c. When done remove from pan.

d. Turn off the stove.

## 6. Poached

a. Gather all needed tools and materials.

b. In a shallow pan, bring 5 to 7 cm (2 to 3 inches) of salted water to the boil.

c. When boiling, reduce the heat to minimum (it should be kept below a simmer while the eggs cook because stronger heat would turn the whites rubber and might cause the egg to stick to the base of the pan) or turn off the heat before adding the eggs. To minimize the spreading of the whites, break the egg directly in the water being careful to open the two halves of the shells and sliding the eggs into the water smoothly.

d. Cover the pan with a tight-fitting lid in order to retain heat.

e. Leave the eggs to cook undisturbed in the water for 3 minutes, then lift off the lid. If the whites are opaque and the yolks covered with a thin, translucent layer of white, the eggs are ready.

 f. Remove the eggs from the pan with a perforated spatula.

 g. Place the eggs immediately in a shallow dish filled with cold water to arrest their cooking. The dish should be big enough to hold all the eggs without crowding.

 h. Lift the eggs out of the water to drain. Trim the edges of the eggs before serving.

## 7. Scrambled

 a. Gather all needed tools and materials.

 b. Break egg into a bowl and beat until frothy.

 c. Set the stove in low Temperature (gently cooking is essential for impeccable scrambled eggs: the lower the heat and the longer the cooking time, the creamier the finished dish will be.)

 d. Grease the pan.

 e. Pour the beaten egg in the pan, stir while adding milk.

 f. Wait till it becomes fluffy.

 g. When done remove from pan.

 h. Turn off the stove.

## 8. Sunny Side-Up

a. Gather all needed tools and materials.

b. Set the stove in low temperature.

c. Grease the pan with small amount of oil.

d. When hot, break one egg into the pan, then add salt (optional).

e. Cover and uncover once in a while.

f. Remove from pan when done.

g. Turn off the stove.

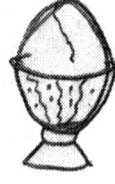

---

**Poached Eggs**

⊛ If you do not have n egg poacher, you can use the rim of jar. Lightly grease the inside of the rim to prevent the egg from sticking. Add a drop of lemon juice to the water to keep the egg whites from spreading.

---

**Freshness of Eggs**

⊛ Fresh eggs will sink in water.

---

**Storing Egg Yolks**

⊛ Egg yolks can be kept fresh for several days with cold water and refrigerating.

---

**Boiled Eggs**

⊛ To prevent boiled eggs from cracking, let is stand on warm water for a while prior to cooking.

⊛ Eggs will not crack if you make a small hole with a needle in the large end of egg before boiling.

⊛ When slicing hard boiled eggs, dip the knife in water periodically to prevent the yolks from crumbling.

## TABLE SETTING

1. **Cover.** Arrangement of china, silverware, napkin and glassware at each place setting. Parts of the cover are dinnerware, glassware, flatware, and linen.

2. **Dinnerware.** Plates of all sizes including dishes, cups, saucers and under liners. This is also known as CHINAWARE.

Examples:

1. Dinner plate
2. Lunch plate
3. Salad or dessert plate
4. Bread and butter plate
5. Cup
6. Soup or salad bowl
7. Dessert bowl
8. Vegetable bowl
9. Soup can
10. Saucer

3. **Flatware.** Refers to knives, forks and spoons, regardless of style or usage. This is also known as SILVERWARE.

Examples:

1. Cocktail fork or oyster fork
2. Salad fork
3. Dinner fork
4. Dinner knife
5. Butter knife
6. Steak knife
7. Iced tea spoon
8. Serving spoon
9. Teaspoon
10. Soup or bullion soup

4. **Glassware.** Glass decanters, pitchers, and all drinking vessels used at the table or bar.

Examples:

1. Small juice glass
2. Large juice glass
3. Water or milk glass

4. Ice tea glass
5. Sherbet glass
6. Parfait glass

5. **Halloware.** Service items of depth or volume including platters, trays and stands.

6. **Linens.** Part of the table setting used to cover table or pipe mouth.

1. Table cloth
2. Napkins

3. Placemat
4. Bibs

Examples:

7. **Underliner.** Extra part of dinnerware placed under service pieces. Examples: dessert bowl or soup cup with underliner.

## ACCESSORIES FOR THE TABLE

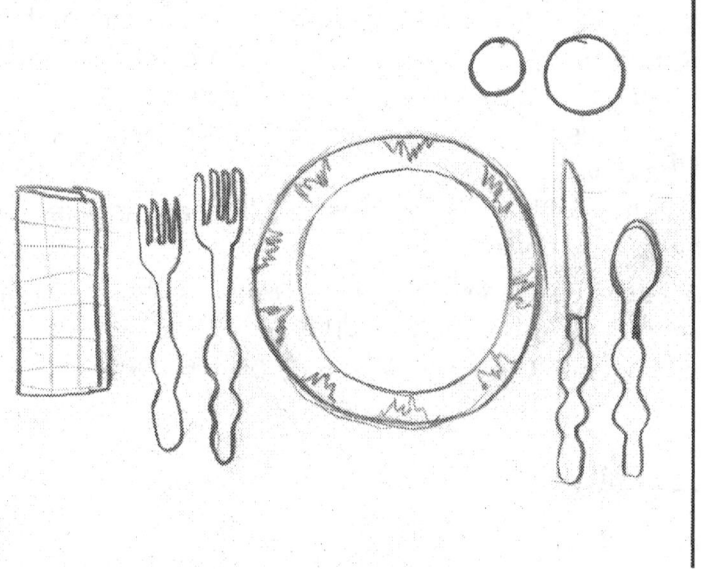

1. Salt and pepper shakers
2. Ashtrays
3. Bread baskets
4. Halloware
   a. Pitcher
   b. Creamers
   c. Sugar bowls
   d. Ice buckets
   e. Tea and coffee sets
   f. Platters
   g. Trays
   h. Bowls
   i Punch bowl

5. Candles
6. Flowers
7. Condiment server
8. Serving pieces
   a. Pastry serve
   b. Serving spoon
   c. Serving fork
   d. Soup laddle
   e. Sugar spoon
   f. Gravy or sauce laddle
   g. Pie or cake serving knife

## BASIC RULES FOR SETTING COVER

1. **Spacious Dining Table.** A spacious dining table is required to accommodate all the family members.
2. **Table Cloth/ Placemats.** The table must be covered with cloth, although placemats have been found practical.
3. **Dinner plate, flatware, beverage ware.** Each cover is completely laid including the dinner plate, the necessary flatware and beverage ware.
4. **Base of Flatware.** Base of all flatware should be even and placed one (1) inch away from the edge of the table.
5. **Knife and spoon.** Knife and spoon are placed on the right side of the cover.
6. **Knife's cutting edge**. Knife's cutting edge should be towards the plate.
7. **Fork.** Fork is placed on the left side of the cover.

8. **Order of flatware.** Flatware is placed in order of use starting from the outside with fork from left, knife and spoon from the right.

9. **Water glass.** Water glass is placed just above the tip of the knife.

10. **Cups and saucers.** Cups and saucers are placed at right side of the plate with the handles towards the edge of the table.

11. **Napkin.** Napkin is placed at the left side of the fork, under the fork, or in the center of the cover.

12. **Platters**. Platters of food with corresponding flatware are placed in the middle of the table on hot pads.

13. **Water Spots on Chinaware, etc.** Always replace china, glassware, and flatware that have water spots or dried foods on them.

14. **Decorations.** Decorations may or may not be used.

## SERVING THE FOOD

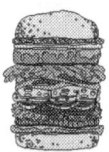

**Food**

- Food is served from the left of the guest and cleared from the right.
- Food being served is placed at intervals on the center of the table.
- The person nearest the dish may start helping himself to it, then passes it on the center of the table.

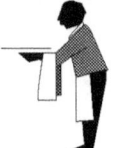

- After each on has been served, the platters are placed back in the middle of the table.
- There is no sequence to which course will be served or eaten first.

**Second Serving**

- When second serving are desired, anyone can help himself for more either by reaching for the dish if he or she is near or by asking for it to be passed.

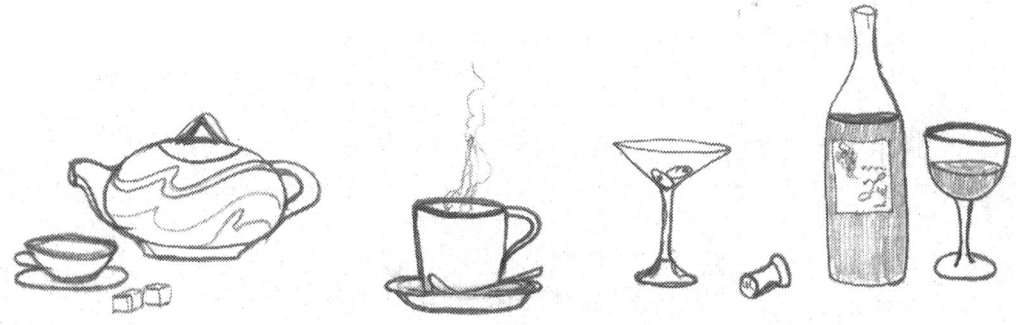

**Beverages**

- Beverages are served and removed from the right of the person eating.

**3-26**

**Dessert**

- ▪ The dessert's course may or may not be on the table at the start. It may be served from the kitchen in individual dishes or from the platter.

## BUSSING OR DISHING OUT

In clearing, platters of food are brought to the kitchen first, then the individual plates, cups, and flatware. If clearing was not done before serving dessert, plates may be piled together on the table and then brought out.

| *Ammonia* |
|---|
| ✿ Cleans clothing, gold, shoes, silver jewelry, ovens, faucets, chrome, diamonds, etc. |

| *Toothpaste* |
|---|
| ✿ Shines jewelry and silverware. |

| *Hairspray* |
|---|
| ✿ Removes various kinds of stains: coffee and tea, lipstick, marker on walls. |

| *Vinegar* |
|---|
| ✿ Cleans appliances, bathtubs, chromes, drains, faucets, garbage disposers, showers, toilet bowels, etc. |

| *Baking Soda* |
|---|
| ✿ Cleans appliances, bathtubs, carpets, china, counters, drains, floors, laundry, marble, pots and pans. |

## 3.5                SPECIAL PROJECT: FOOD COLLAGE

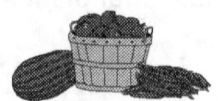

Create a poster using a collage of the four food groups (Bread, Meat, Dairy Products, and Fruits and Vegetables). Make sure that the groups can be distinguished from each other. You may draw, cut and paste, or use actual photos. This assignment is due during the course to receive a 10% bonus mark.

## THE CONCEPT OF SAFE FOOD HANDLING

**3-28**
**10 GUIDELINES IN STORING FRUITS AND VEGETABLES**

1. Keep unripe fruits at room temperature.
2. Store ripe fruits (except pineapple, banana) in a cool place.
3. Place cut lemons, oranges, melons cut-side down in plate or covered container and store in the fridge.
4. Keep fresh berries wrapped in paper in refrigerator and wash shortly before using.
5. Keep left-over berries in tightly covered glass jar in refrigerator.
6. Sort fruits carefully and remove any over ripe fruits.
7. Don't pile soft fruits in storage.
8. Don't store fruits in warm place unless you want to speed ripening.
9. Store potatoes, onions, beets, carrots, and other root vegetables in a cool, dry, well-ventilated area.
10. Keep other vegetables in crisper of refrigerator.

## 5 REMINDERS IN BUYING/SELECTING FRUITS AND VEGETABLES

1. When buying fresh fruits, ensure that the stems are not dried up, but fruits that ripen on the tree, though fresh may have shriveled stems. Vegetables must be free from cuts and bruises and their leaves are fresh, not dried or wilted.

2. The proper selection of vegetables will ultimately result in very tasty and appetizing dishes. Thus, it is important that one must know how to select and prepare vegetables.

3. Buy vegetables which are in season because they are cheaper and in better quality.

4. Choose vegetables which are crisp and bright in color with no signs of decay or rotting.

5. Fresh vegetables cannot be stored for a very long time. Buy only enough and clean or wash before storing.

## 3 TIPS IN BUYING FRESH MEAT

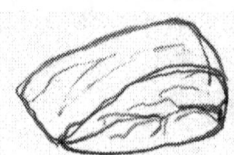

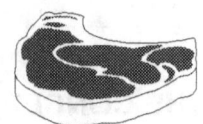

1.     Meat carcass must be compact, firm and plump.
2.     Loin, rib and chuck must be thick, full and moderately fleshed.
3.     Fat covering meat must be fairly smooth and uniformly distributed.

## 4 POINTERS IN SELECTING POULTRY

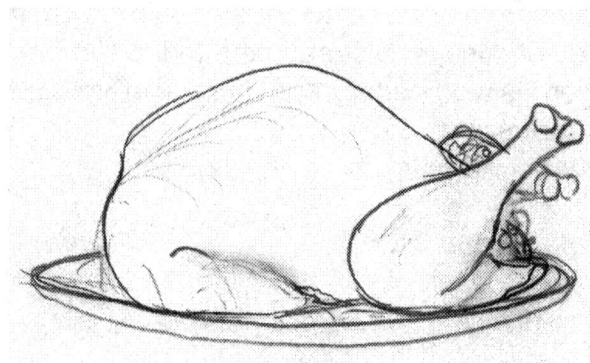

1.     Skin must be smooth and yellow in color.
2.     Breast must be plump.
3.     Thighs must be well developed.
4.     Neck and shanks must be moderately short.

## 5 TIPS IN BUYING FISH

1.     Fresh fish must not have objectionable odor.
2.     Its eyes must be clear, full and right, not dull or sunken (eyes must not be red because this means the fish is no longer fresh).
3.  Its gills must be bright red. Its flesh must be firm and flexible.
4.  The abdomen and belly walls must be intact and free from discoloration.
5.  Fish must be covered with natural slime and have a natural fishy odor.

## 6 SAFETY MEASURES IN FOOD HANDLING

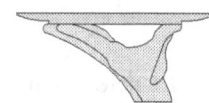

1.  Wash hands before and after.
2.  Wash fruits and vegetables before starting.
3.  Disinfect cutting boards after use.
4.  Thaw meat in the fridge.
5.  Cover left over food individually before storing in the fridge.
6.  Check and label stored foods.

### Non-browning apples or bananas

❀ When peeling a quantity of apples or bananas, place the peeled fruits in a basin of cold, slightly salted water. Otherwise, any juice will also do the trick (grapefruit or lemon juice).

### Buying oranges

❀ The smaller ones are generally sweeter. Look for those that feel heavy for their size and should have a sweet smelling scent.

### In general, when peeling fruits...

❀ Blanch fruits for 45 seconds in boiling water to peel off most skin on fruit

To remove fruit stain from hands..
❀ To remove strawberry or other fruit stains from hands, rub with a paste of cornmeal and lemon juice

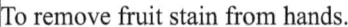

### Buying peppers....

❀ The freshest sweet pepper is one that has a firm and shiny skin.

### Buying cucumbers...

❀ They should be firm and rigid.
❀ To remove the waxy film on the cucumber, rub it with some vinegar.

### Buying potatoes...

❀ They should have a good uniform shape.
❀ Size is important as long as they have a good weight in them.
❀ Look for potatoes that have firm and smooth texture.

# 3.7 SELECTED RECIPES

## 3.7.1 SOUPS

### CANADIAN CHEESE SOUP

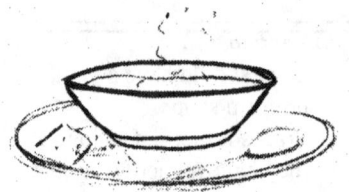

| | | | |
|---|---|---|---|
| 2 | medium carrots, cut in 2.5 cm pieces | 2 | cups (500 ml) water |
| 3 | stalks celery, cut in 2.5 cm pieces | 2 | cups milk |
| ¼ | cup flour | 1 | small onion, quartered |
| 2½ | cups of cheese | 2 | chicken boullion cubes |

Put carrots, celery, onion, and boullion cubes into osterizer blender container. Cover and process 2 cycles at grind until vegetables are finely chopped. Pour into saucepan. Cover and cook until vegetables are tender. Put milk, flour and cheese into blender container. Cover and process at liquefy until mixture is smooth. Stir into vegetable mixture, cook until thickened.

### CREAM OF TURKEY SOUP

½ cup butter
6 tablespoon flour
½ teaspoon salt
¾ cup coarsely chopped cooked turkey

Pinch black pepper
2 cups half and half cream
3 cups turkey or chicken broth

Heat butter in a saucepan. Blend in flour, salt and pepper. Heat until bubbly. Gradually add half and half cream and 1 cup of broth, stirring constantly. Bring to boil, cook and stir 1 to 2 minutes. Blend in remaining broth and turkey. Heat, do not boil. Garnish with grated carrot.

*6 SERVINGS*

### FRENCH ONION SOUP

5 medium onions, sliced (4 cups )
1 tbsp. butter or margarine
1 ½ quarts beef broth

½ teaspoon salt
1/8 teaspoon pepper
cheese croutons

Sauté onions in melted butter in a large saucepan. Cook slowly, stirring until golden (about 10 minutes). Blend in beef broth, Salt and pepper. Bring to boil, cover and simmer 15 minutes. Pour soup into warm soup bowls or crocks. Float a cheese croutons in each bowl of soup.

*6 SERVINGS*

### SEAFOOD CHOWDER

| | | | |
|---|---|---|---|
| 1½ | pounds North Pacific halibut, fresh or frozen | ¼ | cup chopped green pepper |
| 1 | can ( 7½ ounces) Alaska King crab or | 2 | cloves garlic, minced |

| | | | |
|---|---|---|---|
| 2 | package (6 ounces) frozen Alaska crab | ¼ | cup butter or margarine |
| 3 | medium potatoes | 2 | cans (16 ounces each) tomato |
| 1 | large sweet Spanish onion | 2 | cups clam-tomato juice |
| ¾ | cup chopped celery | 1½ | teaspoon salt |
| ¼ | teaspoon thyme | ¼ | teaspoon marjoram |
| 1 | dozen small hard-shell clams | | Snipped parsley |

Defrost halibut, if frozen.  Cut into 1 inch chunks.  Drain canned crab and slice. Or defrost, drain and slice frozen crab.  Pare potatoes and cut into ½ inch  pieces. Peel and thinly slice onion. In a saucepot, sauté onion, celery, green pepper, and garlic in butter. Add tomatoes with liquid, clam-tomato juice, and seasonings.  Cover and simmer for 30 minutes. Add halibut or until halibut and potatoes are done and clam shells open. Add crab and heat  thoroughly. Sprinkle with parsley.  Serve with buttered crusty bread.

*8 SERVINGS*

## SPLIT PEA SOUP

| | |
|---|---|
| 1 pound dried split peas, rinsed | ½ cup sliced celery |
| 1 ½ pounds smoked ham hocks | 2 teaspoons salt |
| 1 cup chopped onion | 6 whole peppercorns |
| 1 bay leaf | 1 ½ quarts water |

Mix all ingredients into an electric cooker. Cover and cook on low heat for 8 to 10 hours. Remove ham hocks and dice meat; reserve ham. Discard bay leaf and peppercorns. Pour soup, about 1 quarter at a time, into an electric blender and blend until smooth. Return soup to cooker.  Put in ham and keep hot until serving time.

*6 TO 8 SERVINGS*

## 3.7.2  MAIN DISHES

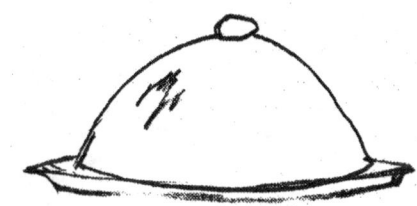

## BEEF POT ROAST

1 beef round rump or chuck roast, boneless (3 ½ pounds)Bouillon or meat broth (about 1 ½ cups)
    3 tablespoons salad oil or  ¼ pound salt pork, diced    1 bay leaf
    2 onions, quartered    2 carrots, cut in pieces
    ½ teaspoon salt    ½ teaspoon coarse pepper
    flour    salt and pepper

Brown the beef in oil. Add ¼ cup bouillon, bay leaf, onions, carrots, salt and pepper, cover and simmer 2 ½ hours, basting with additional bouillon to prevent burning. Sprinkle flour over meat and turn it over. Sprinkle with more flour. If necessary, add more bouillon for the sauce. Cook uncovered for 30 minutes. Serve the pot roast with noodles or potatoes and any kind of vegetables.

*4 SERVINGS*

**Pot Roast with Sour Cream.** Prepare Beef Pot Roast as directed. Add 1 ½ cups sour cream instead of bouillon after flouring the meat. Finish cooking as directed.

**Pot Roast with Sour Cream and Pickles or Mushroom.** Prepare Beef Roast as directed. Add 1 ½ cups sour cream instead of bouillon after flouring the meat. Then stir in 2/3 cup chopped dill pickles or 1 cup sliced mushrooms. Finish cooking as directed.

Arrange all other ingredients in individual mounds in skillet. Top with beef. Cook until vegetables are just tender. Do not stir. Serve immediately with bowls of hot cooked rice.

## CHICKEN WITH RICE

| | |
|---|---|
| 1 broiler-fryer chicken (2 to 3 pounds), cut in pieces | 3 cups hot water |
| ¼ cup fat | 1 cup uncooked rice |
| ½ cup chopped onion | 1 tablespoon minced parsley |
| 1 clove garlic, minced | 1 large tomato, chopped |
| 2 teaspoon salt | ½ teaspoon paprika |
| ¼ teaspoon pepper | ¼ teaspoon saffron |
| 1 bay leaf | |

Rinse chicken and pat dry with absorbent paper. Heat fat in a skillet over medium heat. Add onion and garlic, cook until onion is tender. Remove with a slotted spoon, set aside. Put chicken pieces, skin side down, in skillet. Turn to brown pieces on all sides. When chicken is browned, add tomato, onion, water, rice , parsley and dry seasonings. Cover and cook lower heat about 45 minutes, or until thickest pieces of chicken are tender when pierced with fork.

*6 TO 8 SERVINGS*

## CRUNCHY FRIED CHICKEN

| | |
|---|---|
| 1 cup all purpose flour | ½ teaspoon salt |
| ¼ teaspoon pepper | 2 eggs |
| ½ cup beer | 1 broiler – fryer chicken (2 to 2 ½ pounds), cut up |
| cooking oil | |

Mix flour, salt and pepper. Beat eggs with beer, add to flour mixture. Site until smooth. Dip chicken in battler, coating pieces well. Chill 1 hour. Fry chicken in hot oil ½ to 1 inch deep 15 minutes on one side. Turn, fry on other side 5 to 10 minutes, or until browned and done. Drain on absorbent paper.

*4 SERVINGS*

### COUNTRY FLAVORED CHICKEN HALVES

> 1 packaged 15 minute chicken marinade1 cup water
> 1 broiler – fryer (2 ½ to 3 pounds), cut in half

In a shallow pan, thoroughly blend chicken marinade and water. Place well-drained chicken in marinade, turn, pierce all surfaces of chicken deeply with fork. Marinade only 15 minutes, turning several times. Remove chicken from marinade and arrange skin side up in a shallow ungreased pan just large enough to accommodate the chicken. Bake uncovered, at 425°F from 45 minutes, until thoroughly cooked.

*4 SERVINGS*

### GOLDEN PORK CHOP BAKE

| | |
|---|---|
| 6 pork chops, 1 inch thick | 2 cans (10 ¾ ounces each) condensed golden mushroom soup |
| 2 tablespoons shortening | 1 1/3 cups water |
| ½ cup sliced celery | 1 garlic clove, minced |
| 1 1/3 cups packaged pre-cooked rice | ½ cup chopped tomato |

Brown pork chops on both sides in shortening in a skillet. Remove chops from skillet, drain off excess fat. Sauté celery and garlic in skillet. Combine with remaining ingredients. Spoon into a 2 quart shallow baking dish. Arrange chops on top rice mixture. Cover. Bake at 350°F for 1 hour, or until chops are tender.

*6 SERVINGS*

### HAMBURGER FAVORITES

> 1 ½ pounds ground beef          1 ½ teaspoon salt
> ¼ teaspoon pepper               1 tablespoon fat

Bring out a large, heavy skillet. Mix ground beef lightly with a mixture of salt and pepper. Shape into 6 – 8 patties about ¾ inches thick. Heat fat in skillet. Place patties in skillet and cook over medium heat until brown on one side. Turn the brown side to heat the other side of the patties until brown. Allow 10 to 15 minutes for cooking thick patties and 6 to 10 minutes for cooking thin patties. Remove from skillet to warm serving platter. Garnish with parsley.

*4 TO 6 SERVINGS*

### HEARTY SAUSAGE SUPPER

| | |
|---|---|
| 1 jar (16 ounces) applesauce | 2 tablespoons firmly packed brown sugar |
| 1 can (14 ounces) sauerkraut, drained | 1 can (16ounces) small white potatoes, drained |
| 1/3 cup dry white wine | 1 can (16 ounces) small whole onions, drained |

Mix together applesauce, sauerkraut, wine, and brown sugar. Put into 2 ½ quart casserole. Arrange potatoes and onions around the edge of the casserole. Place sausage in center. Cover. Bake at 350°F for 50 minutes, or until through. Sprinkle with parsley.

*4 SERVINGS*

## *ISLAND STYLE SHORT RIBS*

| | |
|---|---|
| 4 pound lean beef and short ribs | ½ cup soy sauce |
| 1/3 cup sugar | 2 tablespoon vinegar |
| 1 tablespoon vegetable oil | 1 teaspoon ginger |
| ½ teaspoon lemon pepper seasoning | ¼ cup butter or margarine |
| 1 large onion, finely chopped | 2 cups water |

Cut meat from bones, reserve the bones. Trim off as much fat as possible. Cut meat into cubes. Put meat into a bowl. Combine soy sauce, sugar vinegar, oil, ginger, lemon pepper seasoning, and garlic salt. Pour mixture over meat. Cover and refrigerate several hours or overnight. Sauté onion in butter in a skillet. Add onions, marinade, and water. Put into a 2 quart casserole. Top with bones. Bake, covered at 3250F 1 ½ hours. Remove bones and bake, uncovered, for an additional 30 minutes, or until meat is tender. To serve, spoon broth over hot, cooked rice.

*8 SERVINGS*

## *ORANGE-GLAZED PORK LOIN*

| | |
|---|---|
| 1 pork loin roast (3 to5 pounds) | 1 can (6 ounces) frozen orange juice concentrate |
| 3 tablespoons butter | ½ cup water |
| ½ cup lightly packed brown sugar | 2 teaspoons cornstarch |
| 1 cup seeded and halved green grapes | |

Score fat on pork roast at 1 inch intervals. Place roast up on grill directly over dip pan prepared from 3 thickness of heavy aluminum foil. Insert meat thermometer through fat into very center of the meat. Place cover on kettle type grill, adjust dampers, and cook at low heat (approximately 350°F) until meat thermometer registers 170°F (allow 20 to 30 minutes per pound of pork.

For sauce, heat butter in a quart saucepan. Stir in brown sugar. Add orange concentrate and stir until smooth. Remove ¼ cup sauce, stir water into cornstarch. Add gradually to remaining orange juice mixture. Cook, stirring constantly until the mixture thickens. Cook for 8 minutes. Serve hot with pork.

To complete sauce, stir water into cornstarch. Add gradually to remaining orange juice mixture. Cook stirring constantly until thickened. Cook 8 minutes. Serve hot with pork.

*6 TO 12 SERVINGS*

## *POTATO FROSTED MEAT LOAF*

| | |
|---|---|
| 1 ½ pounds ground beef | ½ chopped onion |
| teaspoon salt | ¼ teaspoon pepper |
| 1/8 teaspoon oregano | 2/3 cup quick or old fashioned oats, uncooked |
| 1 egg, beaten | ½ cup milk |
| 2 cups hot mashed potatoes | |

Thoroughly combine all ingredients except mashed potatoes. Pack firmly into an 8 ½ x 4 ½ x 2 ½ inch loaf pan Bake at 350° about 1 hour. Drain off excess fat. Let stand a few minutes, remove from pan. Place on broiler rack. Frost loaf with mashed potatoes. Place under broiler 5 to 7 inches from heat 2 to 3 minutes. Serve immediately.

*8 SERVINGS*

* Four medium sized potatoes will yield about 2 cups mashed potatoes.

## *ROAST CHICKEN WITH POTATOES*

1 chicken (about 4 pounds)
juice of 1 lemon
5 medium potatoes
¼ medium potatoes, pared

salt and pepper to taste
¼ cup butter
1 cup water

Season chicken, inside and out, with salt, pepper, lemon juice, butter and paprika. Place chicken on a rack in a baking in a baking dish. Bake at 350°F about 1 ¼ hours, or until chicken is tender, basting occasionally. After the first of cooking, pour in water, add potatoes and baste with drippings. Turn oven control to 400°F. Remove chicken to a platter and keep warm. Turn potatoes over in a dish. Bake an additional 5 to 20 minutes.

*5 SERVINGS*

## *ROAST STUFFED TURKEY*

1 turkey (6 to 8 pounds)
½ cup melted butter
2 tablespoons butter
½ cup chopped onion

1 package (7 ounces) herb seasoned stuffing croutons
½ cup hot water or chicken broth
½ cup chopped celery
2 tablespoon chopped parsley

Rinse turkey with cold water, pat dry. Turn stuffing croutons into a bowl, add ½ cup melted butter and toss gently. Stir in hot water or broth. Heat 2 tablespoon butter in a skillet. Add celery and onion, cook until tender. Add to bowl with stuffing, and parsley and toss to mix. Spoon stuffing into cavities of bird. Place turkey, breast side up, in a large electric cooker. Insert a meat thermometer in inner thigh muscle. Brush with melted butter. Cover and roast at 3000F until meat thermometer registers 180 to 1850F, about 6 hours.

*6 TO 8 SERVINGS*

## *SHEPERD'S PIE*

1 ½ cups Béchamel Sauce
1 egg beaten
¼ chopped parsley
1 teaspoon thyme
1 teaspoon vinegar
1 teaspoon paprika

1 medium onion, minced
¼ cup fresh cracker crumbs
1 teaspoon salt
¼ teaspoon ground red pepper
1 pound coarsely ground lamb or lean beef
½ cup grated kefalotyl cheese

Combine ¾ cup Béchamel sauce, onion, egg, cracker crumbs, parsley, salt thyme, red pepper and vinegar. Combine sauce with meat, tossing with forks to mix lightly. Spoon mixture into a baking dish. Level top lightly with the back of the spoon. Make an indentation in the center. Bake at 350°F 30 minutes, removing fat as it collects in the indentation. Remove meat from oven when done. Sprinkle with cheese. Cover with potatoes. Sprinkle with paprika. Bake 20 minutes.

4 SERVINGS

## SHRIMP KABOBS

Raw shrimp (about 2 pounds), shelled (leaving on tails) and deveined

12 large pimento stuffed olives

1 inch strips green pepper (using 2 peppers)

1 cup Basic Molasses barbecue Sauce

12 whole mushrooms, cleaned

1 to 2 tablespoons pineapple syrup (optional)

12 large pitted ripe olives

1 tablespoon prepared horseradish

small cooked white onions (16 ounce can, drained)

Thread shrimp, green pepper, onions, mushrooms and olives onto 8 to 10 inch skewers. Combine sauce, horseradish and pineapple syrup, if used. Mix well and brush generously over kabobs. Cook 5 to 6 inches above the hot coals, 5 minutes on each side, brush with the sauce several times during cooking .

*6 KABOBS*


## STANDING RIB OF ROAST BEEF

3-rib (6 to 8 pounds) standing rib roast of beef (have butcher saw across ribs near backbone so it can be removed to make carving easier)

1½ teaspoon salt

1/8 teaspoon pepper

Place roast, fat side up, in a shallow roasting pan. Season with a blend of salt and pepper. Insert meat thermometer so tip is slightly beyond center of thickest part of lean; be sure tip does not rest on bone or in fat. Roast at 300 to 325°F, allowing 23 to 25 minutes per pound for rare, 27 to 30 minutes per pound for medium and 32 to 35 minutes per pound for well done meat. Roast is also done when meat thermometer registered 140°F for rare, 160°F for medium and 170° for well done. Place roast on a warm serving platter. Remove thermometer. For a special treat, serve with Yorkshire Pudding, below.

*8 TO 10 SERVINGS*

Note: A rib roast of beef may be one of three cuts. From the short loin end of the rib section, a first rib roast is cut. This is mostly choice, tender "rib eye" meat. From the center rib roast is cut. It has less "rib eye" meat than the first rib roast and is usually somewhat less expensive. From the shoulder end of the rib section, the sixth and seventh rib roast is cut. It has the least "rib eye" meat and is likely to be least tender of the three. It is usually the least expensive. When purchasing a rib roast, buy not less than two ribs for a standing roast, for a rolled rib roast, buy a 4 pound roast.

**Rolled Rib Roast of Beef.** Follow recipe for Standing Rib Roast of Beef. Substitute rolled beef rib roast (5 to 6 pounds) for the standing rib roast. Roast at 300°F, allowing 32 minutes per pound for rare, 38 minutes per pound for medium and 48 minutes per pound for well done meat.

**Yorkshire Pudding.** Pour ¼ cup hot drippings from roast beef into 11 x 7 x 1 ½ inch baking dish and keep hot. Add 1 cup milk, 1 cup sifted all purpose flour and ½ teaspoon salt to 2 well beaten eggs. Beat with hand rotary or electric beater until smooth. Pour into baking pan over hot drippings. Bake at 400°F 30 to 40 minutes, or until puffed and golden. Cut into squares and serve immediately.

## *SLOPPY JOE*

| | |
|---|---|
| 2 ¼ pounds ground beef | ¼ cup firmly packed brown sugar |
| 2 ½ cups chopped onions | ¼ cup lemon juice |
| 1 cup chopped green pepper | ¼ cup vinegar |
| 1 bottle (14 ounces) ketchup | ½ teaspoon prepared mustard |
| ¼ cup water | 2 teaspoon salt |
| 1 teaspoon pepper | 1 teaspoon Worcestershire sauce |

Brown ground beef, onion and green pepper in a skillet, drain off excess fat. Combine with remaining ingredients. Put into a large oven proof Dutch oven. Bake, covered at 325°F 1 ½ hours. To serve, spoon toasted hamburger buns.

## *SLOW OVEN BEEF STEW*

| | |
|---|---|
| 2 pounds beef stew meat, cut in 1 ½ inch cubes | cups tomato juice |
| 2 medium onions, each cut in eighths | 1/3 cup quick cooking tapioca |
| 3 celery stalks, cut in 1 inch diagonally sliced pieces | 1 tablespoon sugar |
| 4 medium carrots | 2 teaspoons salt |
| 1 bay leaf | 3 medium potatoes |
| ¼ teaspoon pepper | |

Note: Carrots are pared and cut in half crosswise and length wise.
Potatoes are pared and cut ¼ inch thick. Put all ingredients, except potatoes, into a 3 quart casserole. Bake, covered at 300°F for 2 ½ hours. Remove bay leaf and stir in potatoes. Bake, covered an additional 1 hour, or until meat and vegetables are tender.

*8 SERVINGS*

## *STUFFED BAKED FISH*

| | |
|---|---|
| 1 dressed pike, trout or carp (4 to 5 pounds) | salt and pepper |
| 1/3 cup butter or margarine | 2 onions, chopped |
| 3 stalks celery, chopped | 3 apples, cored and chopped |
| 1 tablespoon chopped parsley | 1 cup sliced mushrooms |
| 4 cups dry bread cubes | 2 teaspoon sugar |
| ¼ teaspoon thyme | 2 teaspoon lemon juice |
| 3 eggs | 1 cup water or wine |

Sprinkle cavity of fish with salt and pepper. For stuffing, melt 1/3 cup butter in skillet. Add onion and celery. Stir fry onion until transparent. Add apples, parsley and mushrooms. Stir fry 2 minutes longer. Mix cooked vegetables with bread cubes, sugar, thyme, lemon juice, eggs and water. Blend well. Fill fish cavity with stuffing. Place fish in a roasting pan and drizzle with melted butter. Bake at 3500F about 40 minutes, or until fish flakes easily. Baste occasionally with additional melted butter.

*8 SERVINGS*

### 3.7.3 PIES

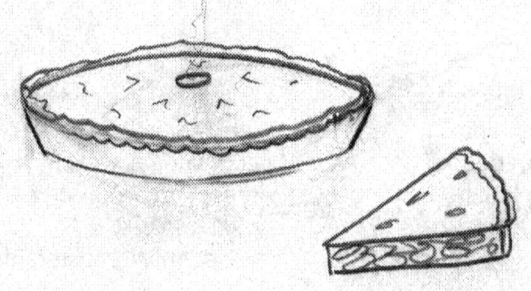

### APPLE PIE

Pastry for crust pie
1 tablespoon lemon juice
3 to 3 ½ tablespoon flour
¼ teaspoon ground nutmeg
2 tablespoons butter or margarine

6 to 8 tart cooking apples
1 cup sugar
1 teaspoon ground cinnamon
1/8 teaspoon salt

Prepare a 9 inch pie shell, roll out remaining pastry for top crust. Set aside. Wash, quarter, core, pare and thinly slice the apples. Turn into a bowl and drizzle with lemon juice. Toss lightly with mixture of sugar, flour, cinnamon, nutmeg and salt. Turn mixture into unbaked pie shell. Dot apples with butter. Complete as for 2 crust pie.

Baked at 4500F 10 minutes, reduces oven temperature to 3500F and bake about 40 minutes, or until crust is lightly browned. Serve warm or cold.

*ONE 9 INCH PIE*

### CREAM PIE

¾ cup sugar
3 tablespoon cornstarch
2 tablespoon flour
1 tablespoon butter or margarine
1 baked 9 inch pie shell or crumb crust

½ teaspoon salt
3 cups milk
3 egg yolks, slightly beaten
1 ½ teaspoons vanilla extract

Mix sugar, cornstarch, flour and salt in a 1 ½ quart saucepan. Stir in one half of the milk, then a blend of remaining milk and egg yolks. Bring to a boil over medium heat, stirring vigorously. Reduce heat, stir and cook about 5 minutes. Turn filling into the pie shell. Chill.

*ONE 9 INCH PIE*

### FRESH BLUEBERRY PIE

Pastry for 2 pie crust
4 teaspoon lemon juice
¼ cup flour
¼ teaspoon ground nutmeg
1 teaspoon grated lemon peel

4 cups fresh blueberries
¾ cup sugar
½ teaspoon ground cinnamon
1/8 teaspoon salt
2 tablespoons butter or margarine

Prepare an 8 inch pie shell, roll out remain pastry for top, crust, set aside. Rinse and drain blueberries. Toss gently with lemon juice, then with a mixture of the sugar, flour, cinnamon, nutmeg, salt and lemon peel. Turn into unbaked pie shell, heaping berries slightly at center, dot with butter. Complete as directed for 2 crust pie.

Bake at 4500F 10 minutes, reduce oven temperature to 3500F and bake 30 to 35 minutes, or until crust is lightly browned. Serve warm or cold.

*ONE 8 INCH PIE*

## FRESH LEMON MERINGUE PIE

**Filling:**

| | |
|---|---|
| 1 ½ cups sugar | 6 tablespoons cornstarch |
| ¼ teaspoon salt | ½ cup cold water |
| ½ cup fresh lemon juice | 3 egg yolks, well beaten |
| 2 tablespoons butter or margarine | 1 ½ cups boiling water |
| 1 teaspoon freshly grated lemon peel | 1 baked 9 inch pastry shell |

**Meringue:**

| | |
|---|---|
| 3 egg whites (at room temperature) | ¼ teaspoon cream of tartar |
| 6 tablespoon sugar | |

For filling, mix sugar, cornstarch and salt together in a 2 to 3 quart saucepan. Using a wire whisk, gradually blend in cold water, then lemon juice, until smooth. Add egg yolks, blending very thoroughly. Add butter. Slowly add boiling water stirring constantly with a rubber spatula.

Over medium to high heat, gradually bring mixture to a full boil, stirring gently and constantly with spatula. Reduce heat slightly as mixture begins to thicken. Boil gently 1 minute. Remove from heat stir in lemon peel. Pour hot filling into pastry shell. Let stand, allowing a thin film to form while preparing meringue.

For meringue, beat egg whites with an electric mixer several seconds until frothy. Add cream of tartar and beat on high speed until egg whites have just lost their foamy appearance. They should bend over slightly when beaters are withdrawn, forming soft peaks.
Reduce speed to medium while gradually adding sugar, about 1 tablespoon at a time. Return to high speed and beat until egg whites are fairly stiff, but still glossy. Soft peaks should be formed when beaters are withdrawn.

Place meringue on hot filling in several mounds around edge of pie. Push meringue to edge of crust to seal. Cover rest of filling by gently pushing meringue towards center of pie.

Bake at 3500F 12 to 15 minutes, or until golden brown. Cool on a wire rack at room temperature away from drafts for 2 hours before cutting and serving.

*ONE 9 INCH PIE*

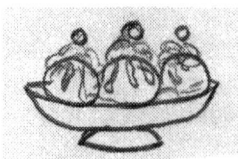

### 3.7.4   OTHER DESSERTS/SWEETS

### *CARROT CUPCAKES*

| | |
|---|---|
| 1 ½ cups sifted enriched all purpose flour | 1 cup sugar |
| 1 teaspoon baking powder | ¾ cups vegetable oil |
| 1 teaspoon baking soda | 2 eggs |
| 1 teaspoon ground cinnamon | 1 cup grated raw carrots |
| ½ teaspoon salt | ½ cup chopped nuts |

Blend flour, baking powder, baking soda, cinnamon and salt. Set aside. Combine sugar and oil in a bowl and beat thoroughly. Add eggs, one at a time, beating thoroughly after each addition. Mix in carrots. Add dry ingredients gradually, beating until blended. Mix in nuts. Spoon into paper baking cup lined muffin pan wells. Bake at 3500F 15 to 20 minutes.

*16 CUPCAKES*

### *CHOCOLATE CHIP COOKIES*

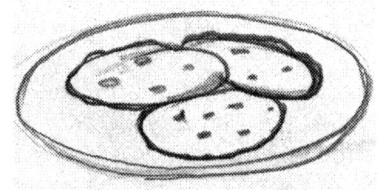

| | |
|---|---|
| 2 ½ cups flour | ½ tsp baking soda |
| ¼ tsp salt | 1 cup brown sugar |
| ½ cup white sugar | 1 cup butter |
| 2 large eggs | 2 tsp vanilla |

Whisk flour, baking soda and salt (dry ingredients).Blend sugar, butter then eggs, then vanilla (wet ingredients).
Mix dry and wet ingredients together. Scoop onto ungreased cookie sheet.

Bake at preheated oven (3000F) for 15 to 20 minutes.

### *CHRISTMAS COOKIES*

| | |
|---|---|
| 3 cups sifted flour | 1 teaspoon baking powder |
| ½ teaspoon salt | ¾ cups butter |
| 1 ½ cups sugar | 2 eggs |
| 1 teaspoon vanilla | food coloring |

Mix flour baking powder and salt. Beat butter, sugar, eggs and vanilla until light and fluffy. Gradually stir in flour mixture. Mix until smooth and well combined. Form dough into a ball and wrap in waxed paper. Refrigerate for several hours or overnight.

Preheat the oven to 3750F. Divide the dough in four parts. Roll out one part at a time. 1/8 inch thick, on a lightly floured surface. Flour cookie cutters and cut out different shapes. Place the cookie on a greased cookie sheet 2 inches apart. Bake 7 to 10 minutes. Decorate with food coloring.

### *OATMEAL COOKIES*

| | |
|---|---|
| 2/3 cup butter or margarine | 1 teaspoon vanilla extract |
| 1 cup firmly packed brown sugar | ½ cup granulated sugar |
| 1 egg | ¼ cup milk |
| 1 cup sifted flour | ¾ tsp salt |
| ½ tsp baking soda | ½ cup walnuts |
| 2 ½ rolled oats | |

Put butter, vanilla extract, sugars, egg and milk in a bowl. Sift flour, salt, and baking soda together. Add to creamed mixture and mix well. Stir in walnuts and oats. Drop by rounded spoonfuls onto greased cookie sheet.

Bake at 4750F 12 to 15 minutes.

*6 DOZEN COOKIES*

---

**Tips for Washing Greasy Dishes**

⊛ If your dishes have that greasy build-up and you're washing them by hand, simply toss a half cup of ordinary baking soda along with the dishes. You should find it cuts the dishwater grease considerably.

⊛ Vinegar is also good to add to your dishwashing water. It is both a mild grease cutter and disinfectant.

⊛ Always start with the cleanest dishes going to the dirtiest ones.

---

**Remove odor!**

⊛ Onion Hands – Believe it or not, you can remove the onion smell on your hands by simply taking hold of a stainless steel spoon and running those hands under cold water. Smell will vanish miraculously!

⊛ Garlic Odor  - When cooking food with a lot of garlic, boil  some distilled white vinegar on the stove at the same time to considerably cut the smell of garlic.

⊛ Freshen up your fridge! Wipe  inside of fridge by wiping periodically with a cloth moistened with vinegar. You can also place a piece of coal on a plastic cup inside the fridge to absorb any unwanted smell.

⊛ For a fresh freezer, just place a loaf for about 3 or 4 nights to get rid of freezer odor.

⊛ For a fresh microwave, place a heat resistant bowl with 3 or 4 slices of lemon and cook for about 3o seconds in the microwave.

# 3.8 QUESTIONS

1. What is the difference between food preparation and food presentation.

2. What are the scientific principles of cooking?

3. List the four food groups.

4. Explain the following coking terminologies:
    a. Garnish :
    b. Peel :
    c. Cube :
    d. Marinade :
    e. Bake :
    f. Fry :
    g. Mince :
    h. Boil :
    i. Roast :
    j. Broil :
    k. Stew :
    l. Chop :
    m. Steam :
    n. Simmer :
    o. Pare :
    p. Grate :
    q. Poach :
    r. Deep Fried:
    s. Grill :
    t. Pressure Cooking:
    u. Braise :
    v. Season :
    w. Grease :
    x. Shred :
    y. Sift :
    z. Dot :

7. Give the eight kinds or ways of cooking egg.

8. What are the components of table setting?

9. List down seven accessories for the table.

10. Enumerate nine examples of halloware.

11. Give seven examples of serving pieces.

12. What are the basic rules for table setting?

13. How do you serve food?

14. How do you clear the table?

15. How do you properly manage fruits and vegetables?

16. How do you select fresh meat from the grocery?

17. How do you select fresh poultry from the grocery?

18. How do you select fresh fish from the grocery?

19. What are some safety measures in handling food?

20. Identify the steps on proper hand-washing procedures.

21. Give 3 examples of soup recipes and its cooking procedures.

22. Give 3 examples of North American main dish recipes.

23. Give 3 examples of pie recipes.

24. Give 3 examples of pastry recipes.

# MODULE
# 4
## CARE OF THE CHILD

### MODULE OBJECTIVES

- State the philosophy of child care and identify the role of caregiver.
- Explain the importance of knowing child development needs and activities.
- Understand the concept of growth and child development.
- Plan to provide for the needs and activities of children.
- Describe the procedure for reporting child abuse.
- Apply the knowledge and skills gained through projects, presentations, and class session and participation.
- The trainee must obtain a passing mark of 85% on critical skills assessed or must repeat until passing mark is attained.

MODULE 4
CARE OF CHILD
TOTAL ALLOTTED TIME: 120 HOURS

TERMINAL OBJECTIVES OF MODULE 4
Upon completion of Module 3, the participant will be able to:
♦ state the philosophy of child care and identify the role of caregiver
♦ explain the importance of knowing child development needs and activities
♦ understand the concept of growth and child development
♦ plan to provide for the needs and activities of children
♦ describe the procedure for reporting child abuse
♦ apply the knowledge and skills gained through projects, presentations and independent study

| TOPICS | SUB-TOPICS TOTAL TIME - 120 hours | LEARNING SITES/TIMES (Classroom) | | |
|---|---|---|---|---|
| | | Theoretical | WORKBOOK FILMS: 4 hrs | *One-on-One Assessment 2 hrs |
| 5.1 Child Care<br><br>5.2 The Importance of Knowing Child Development | 5.1.1. Definition<br>5.1.2 SPICE as an Acronym Social/Physical/Intellectual/Creative/Emotional<br>5.2.1 Concepts of Growth and Development<br>5.2.2 Ages & Stages of Development<br>5.2.3 Basic Development Needs<br>5.2.4 Consequences when Needs are Not Met | 12 hours | Workbook<br>A. The Newborn<br>(0-1 year) | HOW TO:<br>a. lift & hold a baby<br><br>b. bathe an infant<br><br>c. diaper a baby<br><br>d. prepare a formula<br><br>e. bottle feed a baby<br><br>f. burp a baby<br><br>g. dress up a baby<br><br>h. report a child abuse & when |
| 5.3 SPICE Development | 5.3.1 Social Development<br>5.3.2 Physical Development<br>5.3.3 Intellectual Development<br>5.3.4 Creative Development<br>5.3.5 Provider or Emotional Activities | 12 hours | B. The Toddler<br>(1 -2 years)<br><br>C. The Preschooler<br>(2 - 5 years) | |
| 5.4 The Role of the Child Caregiver | 5.4.1 Provider of Social Activities<br>5.4.2 Provider of Physical Activities<br>5.4.3 Provider of Intellectual Activities<br>5.4.4 Creative Development<br>5.4.5 Provider of Emotional Activities | 12 hours | FILMS: 4 hrs.<br>1.Thinking Professionally<br>(30 mins). | |
| 5.5 Health & Safety | 5.5.1 Cleanliness/Sanitation<br>5.5.2 Personal Hygiene & Health<br>5.5.3 House Safety<br>5.5.4 Children 's Diseases | 12 hours | 2. Supporting Family Relations (30 mins) | |
| 5.6 The Value & Stages of Play | 5.6.1 The Value of Play<br>5.6.2 The Stages of Play<br>5.6.3 Toys & Play Equipment | 24 hours | 3.Communicating Through Children (30 mins) | |
| 5.7 Child Abuse/ Management | 5.7.1 The Child Welfare Act of 1984<br>5.7.2 Child Management<br>5.7.3 Approaches to Child Management | 12 hours | 4. Facilitating Play (30 mins) | |
| 5.8 Special Section | 5.8.1 Infant Care (How to: Bathe, Dress, Feed)<br>5.8.2 Nursery Rhymes<br>5.8.3 Games Children Play<br>5.8.4 Children's Favourite Stories<br>5.8.5 Role Playing/Skits/Songs/Poems/Stories | 30 hours | 5. Nurturing thru:<br>*social *physical<br>*creative and<br>*emotional<br>ACTIVITIES | |

*The trainee must obtain a passing mark of 80% on critical skills assessed or must repeat until passing mark is attained.

Text: The Caregiver Resource Manual

# CONTENTS OF MODULE 4

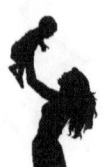

# 4.1 CARE OF THE CHILD

**C**hild Care is the provision of social, physical, intellectual, creative and emotional **(SPICE)** needs and activities to children during their developmental ages ( 0-14 years) and stages.

**T**he Philosophy
of Child Care

It is easy to remember the caregiver's philosophy of child care. It is the provision of **SPICE** needs and activities of children:

**S**ocial

**P**hysical

**I**ntellectual

**C**reative

**E**motional

# 4.2 THE IMPORTANCE OF KNOWING DEVELOPMENTAL AGES AND STAGES

*"No child should be expected to do or behave more than he/she is capable of doing or behaving. We as adults do not have the right to deprive a child of what he can do for and by himself"*

Oftentimes, we think that children are misbehaving when they are only manifesting characteristics of their age and stage of development. Children have yet to develop good judgment and self-discipline (we sometimes expect them to have). As adults, we have to understand the various signs of children's ages and states so we can provide the necessary and appropriate guidance in rearing wise, healthy, and happy children.

Children grow socially, physically, intellectually, creatively, and emotionally. **Growth means Change**. Therefore, we as adults, must know if not learn, what to expect in each stage of development to understand better general children's behavior.

Children follow a general pattern of growth. What does this mean? Simply that most children, at any given age, will be approximately at the same stage of development. Pay attention to the phrase "most children." Just as much we would like to consider the merits of the mentioned statement, we must also remember that children are individuals and individuality counts.

## 4.2.1  Stages of Development

| STAGE | DESCRIPTION |
|---|---|
| Defining Stage | The first 6 years of life |
| Refining Stage | Kindergarten - Junior High |
| Specializing Stage | Security/Stage - Income |
| Fulfillment Stage | Retirement |

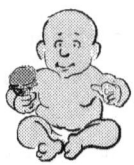

## 4.2.2  Child Development

### Concept of Growth and Development

Human development starts in the womb. A person undergoes growth and development as he goes through the cycle of life.

| | |
|---|---|
| *Growth* | refers to the quantitative changes or increases in size. Everything in us becomes larger physically. |
| *Development* | refers to qualitative changes. It is a progressive series of orderly and coherent changes. |
| *Progressive* | signifies that changes are directional-that they lead forward. |
| *Orderly and Coherent* | means that there is a definite relationship between a given stage and the stages which precede it. |

## 4.2.3  Ages & Stages of Child Development (0-14)

| STAGE | AGE |
|---|---|
| Infant | 0-18 Months |
| Toddler | 19 Months-2 ½ Years |
| Pre-Schooler | 2 ½- 6 Years |
| Schooler | 6-14 Years |

## 4.2.4 THE BASIC DEVELOPMENTAL NEEDS OF CHILDREN

1. The Need for Emotional Development.
2. The Need to be Safe.
3. The Need to have Self-Worth.
4. The Need to Express Self and Feelings.
5. The Need for Success.
6. The Need for Dependence and Independence.
7. The Need to Belong and Get Along.
8. The Need for Social Development.
9. The Need for Physical Development.
10. The Need for Intellectual Development.
11. The Need for Creative Development.

## 4.2.5 CONSEQUENCES WHEN BASIC DEVELOPMENTAL NEEDS ARE NOT MET

*A child* who has never felt safe, has and will never learn to trust his world, and therefore can never learn to be independent.

*A child who doesn't know how things work in this world, or doesn't have the language to express himself, is not able to feel good about himself, for he won't be able to do things.*

*A child who doesn't learn to develop social skills, nor learn the give and take of living with others, cannot find out more about his world or learned new things, for his fear of people will hinder him.*

*A child who is hungry, malnourished, or in poor health, is unable to learn.. he/she can only survive.*

*Therefore, no single need of a child can be neglected, for they are all linked together.*

*It is our responsibility as caregivers (parents, teachers, providers and homemakers) to ensure that while the children remain with us, each of their SPICE needs are met.*

## PLANNING TO MEET THE NEEDS OF CHILDREN
### *OVERVIEW*

- A balance of activity and rest.
  *Ex:  playing outdoors and reading*
- A balance of individual and group activities
  *Ex:  watching TV and playing hide and seek*
- Establishing routines for toileting, resting, and eating which encourage health habits and provide children the security of a well-ordered and planned sequence of events.
  *Ex:  washing before each meal, eating, and resting after eating*
- Providing large blocks of time which allow children to make choices and to explore their environment.
  *Ex:  going for a nature walk before making them come inside                        and once inside, to entertain and satisfy questions and                            observations*
- For older children (school age), a balance of free time, active play and educational activities. Flexibility to take advantage of special activities of occurrences and to keep children from feeling pressured.
  *Ex:  going to the park, mall, celebrating birthdays*

## 4.2.6  Beyond 3 Years and Before Puberty Age

The role of parents/caregiver changes from physical care to controlling behavior of a child. **Socialization** takes place in which a child assimilates the norms and standards set by the society. Parents guide children when norms and standards are violated. Socialization is critical in the child's assuming gender roles, relating with peers, controlling oppression and in developing helpful behaviors.

---

### *SPICE Development Overview*

Children are classified according to their age as:

| | |
|---|---|
| **Infant** | **0-18 months** |
| **Toddler** | **19 months - 2 ½ years** |
| **Pre-schoolers** | **6 years-14 years** |

Before reaching the age of 5 years, development of fine motor skills are exhibited by a child. **Fine motor skills** involve the use of smaller muscular groups which are used in grasping, throwing, catching, and writing.

**Gross Motor Skills** are developed after 5 years old and make use of large areas of body needed in walking, running, jumping, swimming and the like.

An individual's creativity is rooted in his past experiences. Hence, a person's attitudes, values, social interaction, and other behaviors during the basic years of life are essential to creativity.

Being social and creative starts when individual is only a child wherein he/she continuously experiments and discovers new things and situations.

Play is important in enhancing *SPICE* development because explanation and exploration through plays subject the child in social and natural reinforcements.

Social and natural reinforcements assist the individual to increase creativity. Social praises when producing a novel idea or solution stimulates the person to go on reaching. Natural reinforcements as meeting new people, going to new places, trying out new procedures, systems, theories, etc., enhance the person's desire to think, to be more creative and productive.

---

# *SPICE*
## DEVELOPMENT CHARTS


Note:  The next four pages show the development ages and stages
including SPICE profile of children.

## 4.2.7  THE TWO YEAR OLD

### SPICE Development Chart

| SOCIAL | PHYSICAL | INTELLECTUAL | CREATIVE | EMOTIONAL |
|---|---|---|---|---|
| - Still likes to play alone.<br>- Interested in playing with others, not totally involved.<br>- Beginning to develop interest in playing with others.<br>- When playing with others, often argues over toys.<br>- Sharing and operating is difficult<br>- Asks adults when he wants something from another child.<br>- Do not pressure them to be involved or participate.<br>- Stay close by to give support and help manage social situations.<br>- Give warm and caring support and redirect attention from conflict situations. | - Very active, and when tired is irritable or restless.<br>- Jumps, walks, runs and toddles.<br>- Can also clap hands and kick a ball.<br>- More small muscle develop-ment.<br>- Can handle such small objects as crayons, but cannot button, zip and take care of self.<br>- Use many rest activities, such as finger plays and music activities.<br>- Provide activities such as bean bag tossing and other large muscle activities.<br>- Avoid small muscle activities, however, replace with stacking and sorting. | - More language development.<br>- Can put two or three words together into a sentence.<br>- Says no often, even when he doesn't mean to.<br>- Is aware of parents or primary caregivers.<br>- Thinking is simple and direct, cannot deal with abstract concepts.<br>- Can make simple choices.<br>- Has short attention span (two or three minutes).<br>- Children move from one activity to another.<br>- Curious and enjoys repetition.<br>- Cannot reason or make sound judgments.<br>- Teaching activities and discussions must be simple.<br>- Learns best through involvement and repetition.<br>- Vary the activities to choose<br>- Do not leave alone<br>- Take safety precautions because can easily get themselves into situation without considerations of safety<br>- Listen to them and give opportunities for speaking | - Music is an excellent stimulus, however, simple.<br>- Paddycake and nursery rhymes are best.<br>- Large hard covered books, or touch books are great.<br>- Big and bright toys seem to be best suited.<br>- At this stage repetition or parotting of words and activities are easier for the child to mock.<br>- Activities that involve large motor skills.<br>- Large finger painting, water play and dolls or cars with mocking sounds.<br>- Be patient because the child's attention span is minimal.<br>- Choose or set up a learning area and make it fun, colorful and interesting.<br>- The child's environment of play and learning is important.<br>- Choose well lit and bright open areas. | - carefree, has no regard for time<br>- responds warmly, loving and affectionate .<br>- is dependent on adults.<br>- Likes to be close to mother.<br>- Emotional outbursts are a way of letting you know how he feels, of getting what he wants immediately, and of showing anger and frustration.<br>- Moods change quickly or swing like a pendulum.<br>- Likes independence but lacks the skills to be left alone.<br>- Be patient, tolerant, and give lots of praise.<br>- Don't be afraid to hug.<br>- Encourage him to be self-sufficient, however, offer lots of support and help when needed. |

## 4.2.8  THE THREE YEAR OLD

## SPICE Development Chart

| SOCIAL | PHYSICAL | INTELLECTUAL | CREATIVE | EMOTIONAL |
|--------|----------|--------------|----------|-----------|
| - Is centered, sharing is difficult.<br>- Happily plans and works by himself.<br>- Beginning to play with others, but does not engage in much cooperative play with others.<br>- Prefers to be close to adults particularly family, because they give him security.<br>- Use activities that encourage the child to learn to share, wait his turn and cooperate with others.<br>- Develop a close relationship with each child and plan activities that focus on the family.<br>- Build attitudes of care and understanding toward the family and its members.s | - Walks and runs, but coordination still not well developed.<br>- Large muscle development.<br>- Likes doing things with his hands, but may be awkward or messy because of lack of small muscle development.<br>- Use rest activities that give opportunities for large muscle development and coordination such as jumping, skipping, walking or bending. Provide large equipment such as pictures, drawing paper, or crayons.<br>- Avoid puzzles that are too hard and become frustrating.<br>- Plan simple art activities, that follow with easy clean up. | - Has short attention span. Cannot deal with abstract ideas.<br>- Is imaginative- loves to pretend. Likes to become involved in finger plays, and musical and dramatic activities.<br>- Language is rapidly developing. Likes to talk and learn new words.<br>- Often develops misunderstandings. Likes stories and songs.<br>- Alternate between quiet and lively activities. Encourage participation. Present ideas simply and concretely. Use visual aids to clarify lesson objectives.<br>- Let children ask questions and respond to ideas within lessons. Interact<br>- Involve children in group activities and role play.<br>- Use stories and songs in the lesson to teach. | - Creating things at this stage is also part of a self-esteem reinforcement. "See what I can do" stage and my want to repeat over and over.<br>- Small finger activities such as beading or string paint or block stacking can be started with large objects.<br>- Playing house or cars. Doing things adults do becomes important. Puppet shows, helping around the house and doing the chores are encouraged.<br>- The child may sit to watch part of an educational show such as Fred Penner or the Elephant Show.<br>- Have crafts planned prior to child involvement.<br>- Learning through music. | - Is anxious to please adults and is dependent on their approval, care and praise.<br>- May strike out emotionally at situations or persons when there is troublesome feelings, fears or anxieties. May cry easily.<br>- Is sensitive to the feelings of others. Developing some independence and self-reliance.<br>- Give approval- facial and verbal responses.<br>- Avoid negative remarks about the child. Offer care, understanding and patience. Help him work out his own emotions.<br>- Encourage him to do things for himself. |

## 4.2.9  THE FOUR YEAR OLD

### SPICE Development Chart

| SOCIAL | PHYSICAL | INTELLECTUAL | CREATIVE | *EMOTIONAL* |
|---|---|---|---|---|
| - Is still dependent on family. Is more cooperative in his play with others.<br>- Loves to pretend, dramatize, and role play.<br>- May still be physically aggressive, however, is beginning to talk through.<br>- Maybe bossy, impolite or stubborn, as well as cooperative and friendly.<br>- Is learning to share, accept rules and take turns.<br>- Lessons focus on the family.<br>- Give ample opportunity to play with others. Also, reinforce positive social behavior without punishing or scolding. | - Is very active. Moves quickly and lives in a hurry. Uses large muscle to skip, jumps, race and throw ball.<br>- Is sometimes physically aggressive.<br>- Utilize many large muscle activities. Vary activities. Alternate between quiet and lively activities such as stories, songs, games and rest activities.<br>- Help him to learn to control his own behavior and to be responsible for his actions. | - Can reason a little, but still has many misconceptions.<br>- Loves learning new words, playing with words, and talking. Uses fairly complex sentences and asks many questions.<br>- May have trouble separating from fantasy.<br>- Learns through the sense of taste, touch, sight, smell and hearing.<br>- Is curious. Attention span is still short. His art work indicates his feelings.<br>- Give aid in separating fact from fantasy.<br>- Include many sensory experiences in teaching.<br>- Use real objects and actual experiences.<br>- Provide opportunities for exploring and investigating the world around him.<br>- Encourage visual and physical lessons. | - Creativity through role play, TV stories.<br>- Interacting in group settings and inventing certain characters.<br>- Making up stories however, stories lacking direction and structure.<br>- Knowing family members' names. Counting. Remembering parts of stories, songs nursery rhymes, also favorite songs.<br>- Help with some cooking and setting the table, etc. | - Often tests people to see whom he can control. Is boastful, especially about self and family.<br>- Maybe agreeable one minute and quarrelsome or cranky the next.<br>- Has growing confidence in self and the world.<br>- Is beginning to develop some fears and feelings of insecurity.<br>- Establish limits and adhere to them. |

## 4.2.10 THE FIVE YEAR OLD

### SPICE Development Chart

| SOCIAL | PHYSICAL | INTELLECTUAL | CREATIVE | EMOTIONAL |
|---|---|---|---|---|
| - Is more sure of himself and generally more dependable.<br>- Plays well with other children however, can also play by himself (and he chooses one type of play).<br>- When by himself, may amuse himself by skipping or drawing.<br>- Enjoys special outings and abides by going out rules.<br>- Also may be helpful to others and sympathetic.<br>- Will ascertain right from wrong with social behaviors- i.e. (Don't scream in buildings but rather uses inside voices).<br>- A constant reminder of rules and also test rules to border line. | - Large muscle coordination, continues to improve. He can skip, turn somersaults and hop even on one foot.<br>- His small muscle permits him to cut, paste and glue. He may tie his shoes.<br>- Enjoys going on climbers at the park. Swings, running races, and challenging friends to race.<br>- At this stage, daily large muscle release is necessary to let off steam. For outside and inside fun, he now has his one favorite activity.<br>- Games involving exercise are challenging. For example, "Red Rover", "Mother, May I", "Hide and Seek." | - He is very serious when he asks "What is that for?" or " How does this work?" Also, will try to make up his own answers as part of Problem Solving.<br>- He can count to 50, may know his alphabet. May spell his name or start to print and may read the odd word.<br>- Is more reliable and independent and wishes to do more chores now that he thinks, "He is a BIG PERSON NOW", (making associations he could do more this year now that he is five as last year when he was four).<br>- More responsibility is what he wants. So in moderation and supervised allow his intellect to expand. | - He can create pictures from memory from early stories, TV shows or favorite activity.<br>- Pictures are becoming more structures with more color and color variety.<br>- Will cut boxes or make houses for dolls or cars.<br>- More of a verbal role play with "I am the Mommy and this is what I do".<br>- More insight of how things work and the world around him.<br>- Pretend play, arrange chairs to make a bus or train.<br>- The child will express his need for creativity.<br>- Listen, more one on one while the child is drawing and asking questions of the child. | - He has now the vocabulary to express his feelings of love-anger-frustration.<br>- Also this is a period where testing of his emotions are quite common. "I don't like you" or "You can't be my friend."<br>- He will often demand what another child is playing with as a right.<br>- Because one child wants an object he will think that the other child has had it long enough, even though he has played with the object for a very short time. The result is often a quarrel.<br>- Proper direction of free play and structured play has to be supervised. |

# 4.3 THE ROLES OF THE CAREGIVER

This section deals with the identification of caregiver's role expectations and children's change of behaviors through developmental activities.

## 4.3.1 PROVIDER OF SOCIAL ACTIVITIES

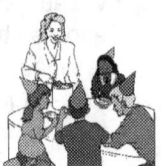 ***Social needs*** are characterized by a child's need to behave and interact positively with members of his family, his caregiver, friends, and learned acceptable behavior.

| Caregiver's Role Expectations | Children's Expected Behaviors |
|---|---|
| ■ Models acceptable and appropriate social behavior. | ■ Develop harmonious and positive relationship with family members, caregiver, and adults. |
| ■ Plans daily activities that meet the child's social needs as an individual and as a member of a group. | ■ Behave appropriately in a group. |
| ■ Provides activities in a setting that encourages social interaction among playmates, members of the family, and others (adults). | ■ Share, play, and cooperate with others. |
| ■ Offers activities that enhance the child's feeling of respect, sharing, acceptance, and caring among peers and adults. | ■ Appreciate, accept, and respect the needs of others. |
| | ■ Tolerate the behavior of others. |
| | ■ Accept majority's decision. |
| ■ Ignores behaviors which are not socially enhancing and reinforces those which are. | ■ Resolve conflicts and disagreement with others. |

## 4.3.2  PROVIDER OF PHYSICAL ACTIVITIES

The child's **physical needs** are characterized by the growth and development of large and small muscles and the child's perceptual skills.

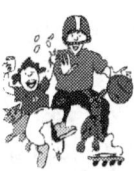

| Caregiver's Role Expectations | Children's Expected Behaviors |
|---|---|
| ■ Plans active and physical activities to meet the child's physical needs.<br><br>■ Provides activities, both indoor and outdoor.<br><br>■ Plans and provides nourishment, rest, varied small activities that stimulate the development of senses. | ■ Develop simple bodily movement and skills such as balance, stability, rhythm, and coordination.<br><br>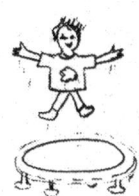 ■ Develop large muscles skills through activities such as running, climbing, dancing, skipping, crawling, exercising.<br><br>■ Develop small muscles through activities such as drawing, painting, scooping, threading, printing, cutting and pasting.<br><br>■ Develop perception through activities involving the five senses, identification of body parts, directional awareness, and exercising body parts, stimulating the senses. |

## 4.3.3  PROVIDER OF INTELLECTUAL ACTIVITIES

**Intellectual needs** of a child are characterized by the need to acquire and use language, learn, explore and experiment with the environment and the need to express opinions and make decisions.

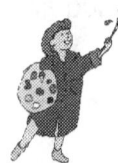

| Caregiver's Role Expectations | Children's Expected Behaviors |
|---|---|
| ▪ Plans activities to meet the child's intellectual needs.<br><br>▪ Provides activities that enhance the child's thinking and reasoning skills.<br><br>▪ Includes activities that stimulate the senses.<br><br>▪ Stimulates the child's appreciation of arts, music and literature. | ▪ Develop language skills by using words and sounds in a variety of ways, following directions, observing and imitating models.<br><br>▪ Develop thinking and reasoning skills through questioning, providing simple accounting of what has been observed or experienced, making use of the five senses, solving puzzles and everyday problems.<br><br>▪ Develop listening skills by caring out simple instructions, listening and repeating <br><br>what has been heard, listening and appreciating songs, music, educational TV shows and cartoons, singing, telling stories, and inventing jokes. |

## 4.3.4  PROVIDER OF  CREATIVE DEVELOPMENT
### 4-8

***Creative needs*** include the development of  a creative mind and body. The process of development of a creative mind involves exposure to experiences of exploration, discover, inventory, observation, creation and experimentation. The process of development leading to a creative body involves exposure to music, drama, the arts and artistic expressions (talent, acquired).

| Caregiver's Role Expectations | Children's Expected Behaviors |
|---|---|
| ▪ Plans activities that stimulate creative thinking and expressions.<br>▪ Provides opportunities and first hand experiences in music, drama, arts, crafts and literature.<br>▪ Encourages questions, explorations, creation and experimentation.<br>▪ Accentuates the ways and means of obtaining a creative product (process)rather than the product itself. | ▪ Develop creative thinking in the form of questions, sensible answers, solutions, expression of imagination, ideas.<br>▪ Use various sensory perceptions in expressing self(pretend, fantasize, imagine, role play)<br>▪ Create, display, discuss and experiment with concrete objects made with hands. |

## 4.3.5  PROVIDER OF EMOTIONAL ACTIVITIES

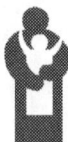 *Emotional needs* are characterized by the need to feel loved, protected, accepted and respected.

| Caregiver's Role Expectations | Children's Expected Behaviors |
|---|---|
| ▪ Plans activities that meet the emotional needs of the child.<br>▪ Provides a place in which the child can feel loved, understood and accepted.<br>▪ Develops activities that enhance the child's self-worth.<br>▪ Creates opportunities where the child can experience various emotions and feelings and that these feelings are recognized and accepted.<br>▪ Provides opportunities where the child can be aware of the difference between feelings(e. g. anger)and negative behavior (breaking things). | ▪ Express feelings appropriately.<br>▪ Learn and understand the difference between feelings and negative behaviors.<br>▪ Use coping mechanisms.<br>▪ Take part in activities that are success oriented and self-worth enhancing. |

Children should always be considered as helpless prey to numerous illnesses and diseases. Safeguarding the child from such disorders must be the primary concern of every caregiver. To do this, the caregiver must start orienting the child on the merits of having a healthy and safe environment and the ways the child can contribute to achieve such conditions.

**4-11**

**4-12**

### Cleanliness and sanitation of surroundings.

The presence of disease-causing bacteria is largely rooted on dirty surroundings. The caregiver must see to it that every area of the house and all its accessories are dirt free and disinfected, especially the kitchen, the washrooms, the play areas, and the child's bedroom.

### Concern for personal hygiene and health.

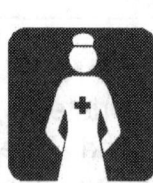

At an early age, the child must be exposed to the importance of a clean body to avoid sickness and diseases. He must be helped in developing the habit of bathing, washing of hands, brushing of teeth, correct use of toilet, and the like .also, the child must be oriented on the essence of seeing a doctor or dentist regularly, eating the right food at the right time and taking appropriate medicines.

### Maintenance of a safe house.

One major responsibility of a caregiver is to see to it that the house is free from all possible sources of diseases and illnesses.

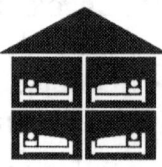

## 4.4.1  TIPS TO CHILD-PROOF THE HOUSE

The following are tips to child-proof the house:

*Hazardous products.*
Keep all hazardous products (poisons, drugs, household cleaning and cooking products)out of reach of children.

*Medicines.*
1. Dispose of all unused medicines and empty containers. Call the nearest pharmacy for advice.
2. Always leave drugs and household products in their original containers.
3. Do not remove labels and instructions on how to take medicines and how to use certain household products.
4. Never give medication to children by referring to it as candy. Say medicine.

*Food.*
1. Never use food or drink containers for storing hazardous products.
2. Do not eat food that may no longer be safe. If in doubt, throw it away.

*Poisonous house plants.*
Know poisonous house plants. They don't belong in the house no matter how attractive or decorative they look.

*Ways poison can enter the body.*
There are four ways in which poison can enter the body. The poison can be swallowed, inhaled, injected or absorbed.

## 4.4.2  CHILDREN'S DISEASES

The following are some important reminders to a caregiver in dealing with children's diseases:

*Determining communicable diseases.*
The caregiver must be able to detect different communicable diseases which affect many people. He/she should be familiar with their symptoms, incubation periods and prevention. The child or patient's comfort must also be taken into account when he/she is suffering from illnesses. It is always better to consult the physician for advice.

### *Handling emergency situations.*

A caregiver must be able to respond to emergency situations. As such he/she must be ready with a list of emergency centers, their addresses and telephone numbers within the community or city. He/ she must be familiar with describing the situations that need immediate attention.

# 4.5 THE VALUE AND STAGES OF PLAY

## 4.5.1 THE VALUE OF PLAY

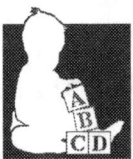

The child grows and learns through play.
Toys are his valuable tools.
It is his characteristics to explore endlessly through various kinds of play.
As he matures and understand the world around him,
play and his daily activities become closer and closer to reality.
Play changes from exploration and experimentation to the use of developing skills
in his attempts to accomplish more complicated and responsible tasks and activities.

***Examples:***
*Playing with younger children becomes a child care job that pays.*
*Riding a bike now becomes a transportation to school.*
*Helping deliver flyers becomes a real good paying job.*
*Helping mother cook becomes a first paying job at McDonalds.*

## 4.5.2 STAGES OF PLAY

These four stages of play describe the way children play games:

**STAGE 1      (1-3 years)**
The child behaves as though there were no rules. He actually knows no rules.

**STAGE 2      (5-7 years)**
The child thinks he is following rules but in reality he is making up his own rules. His play behavior is beginning to emerge, however.

**STAGE 3      (5-11 years)**
The child plays in a seriously social manner. Rules are mutually and rigidly adhered to by all players. Rules are never changed.

**STAGE 4      (11-12 years)**
The child has a complete understanding of the purpose and origin of rules. They are occasionally modified in the course of playing each game

## 4.5.3  TOYS & PLAY EQUIPMENT (AGES&STAGES)

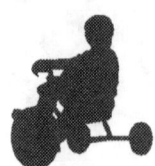 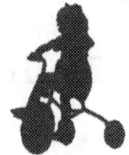

*Toys that encourage sharing*

### Large muscle play materials

climbing apparatus (yard or playground)          bikes
objects for crawling, jumping, riding, running, sliding          jumping ropes
blocks to stack, nest, sort, carry and build with          sorting  toys/push  and  pull
toys

### Role play materials

dolls, puppets, stuffed toys          house appliances toys (iron, plates, etc.)
vehicle toys          hats, costume jewelry
activity sets          adult dresses

### Books and story materials/creative toy materials

cut and paste materials          tape recorder          picture books
fairy tales          story books          play dough
paint, brushes, crayons          large papers          puzzles
construction toys          mix and match toys   lego
beads          origami          building blocks

# 4.6                             CHILD ABUSE

## 4.6.1  THE CHILD WELFARE ACT OF 1984

*Section 1:*

(2)  For the purposes of this Act, a child is in need of protective services if there are reasonable and probable grounds to believe that the survival, security or development of the child is endangered because of any of the following:

    a)  the child has been or there is substantial risk that the child will be physically injured or sexually abused by the guardian (includes parent) of the child.

    b)  the child has been emotionally injured by the guardian of the child;

    c)  the guardian of the child has subjected the child to or is unable or unwilling to protect the child from cruel and unusual treatment or punishment;

(3) For the purposes of this Act,

    a)  a child is emotionally injured

        i)  if there is substantial and observable impairment of the child's mental or emotional functioning that is evidenced by a mental or behavioral disorder, including anxiety, depression, withdrawal, aggression or delayed development, and

        ii)  there are reasonable and probable grounds to believe that the emotional injury is the result of:

            A)  rejection
            B)  deprivation of affection or cognitive stimulation
            C)  exposure to domestic violence or severe domestic disharmony
            D)  inappropriate criticism, threats, humiliation, accusation towards the child or
            E)  the mental or emotional condition of the guardian of the child or chronic alcohol or drug abuse by anyone living in the same residence as the child;

    b)  a child is physically injured if there is substantial and observable injury to any part of the child's body as a result of the non-accidental application of the force or an agent to the child's body that is evidenced by a laceration, a contusion, an abrasion, a scar, a fracture or other bony injury, a dislocation, a sprain, hemorrhaging, the rupture of discus, a burn, a scald, frostbite, the loss or alteration of consciousness or physiological functioning or the loss of hair or teeth;

    c)  a child is sexually abused if the child is inappropriately exposed or subjected to sexual contact, activity or behavior.

*Section 3:*
(1)  Any person who has reasonable and probable grounds to believe and believes that a child is in need of protective services shall forth with report the matter to a director (of Child Welfare).
(4)  No action lies against a person reporting pursuant to this section unless reporting is done maliciously or without reasonable and probable grounds for the belief.
(5)  Any person who fails to comply with subsection (1) is guilty of an offence and liable to a fine of not more than $2000 and in default of payment to imprisonment for a term of not more than 6 months

*Julie V. Kallal*

## 4.6.2  CHILD MANAGEMENT/POSITIVE DISCIPLINE

A positive approach to managing children is highly recommended. To use such an approach, it is essential to reinforce or praise desirable behaviors and to ignore, where possible, undesirable behaviors.

If a situation occurs where there is deliberate destruction of property, or more importantly where child safety is at stake, do the suggested example:

| *Example: When one child is hurting another* |
|---|
| **To do:**  I will remove the offender from the situation for a short TIME OUT. At the same time, it is important that I let the child know verbally that such behavior is unacceptable. *Say: "I cannot let you hurt Tony, that hurts him."* More importantly, when the child has calmed down, I should show him an alternate appropriate behavior. |

The positive approach to child management also helps to protect the child's self-image by focusing on the behaviors rather than the person or personality of the child.

### POLICY #1: Spanking or Shaking of Any Kind is Not Permitted Nor Used by Me

**Child Abuse**

An abused child is one who needs protection for any reason whatsoever. Research and studies indicate that the child abusers (it takes all kinds of people) tend to repeat their own childhood experiences (when they have been abused in one way or another) inventing their frustrations, anger or helplessness in dealing with their problems in life. Likewise, studies indicate that intervention followed by treatment is preferable to criminal action because this process helps maintain the natural family setting of the child.

Child abuse takes many forms:

A ***Neglected Child***  is one who is malnourished, denied medical care, has been abandoned for long periods of time, or has been kept unlawfully from attending school. This child may appear dirty, tired, irritable, hungry and in need of medical care or attention.

A ***Sexually Abused Child***  is one who has been physically and sexually ill-treated.

A ***Battered Child***  is an extreme case of a child abuse, and the child is in need of protection from physical harm.

130

A *Psychologically Abused Child* is one who has been constantly yelled at or criticized and whose self- concept or self esteem has been damaged.

**POLICY #2: I Will Not Permit Nor Allow Child Abuse of Any Kind**

## 4.6.3 APPROACHES TO CHILD MANAGEMENT

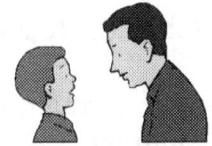 The caregiver shall ensure that the discipline used agrees with that of a kind, firm and just parent. The parent(s) must discuss approaches in dealing with their children behavior and the preferred method of disciplining the child. If the parent(s) do not discuss discipline approaches, then the caregiver must take the initiative.

| Acceptable Approaches to Discipline |
|---|
| The following suggests acceptable approaches to positive discipline:<br>    1. Setting limits.<br>    2. Setting standards of behavior.<br>    3. Providing choices.<br>    4. Providing explanations.<br>    5. Confirming that the child understands.<br>    6. Being firm (but) flexible.<br>    7. Recognizing individual differences  (age, needs, experience).<br>    8. Ignoring most negative behavior.<br>    9. Using alternative when behaviors cannot be ignored.<br>    10. Time out and reverse time out.<br>    11. Rapport.<br>    12. Desensitization. |
| Unacceptable Approaches to Discipline |
|     1. Parent Muscle.<br>      ▪ Spanking, nagging, pinching, screaming, threatening, shaking.<br>    2. Physical Restraint. |

## 4.6.4  INDICATORS OF CHILD ABUSE

| **Some typical signs of a child abuse** |
|---|
| 1.  **Bruises.** Visible marks such as bruises, welts, burns scars and fractures. |
| 2.  **Tiredness, irritability.** The child may be tired, uneasy, irritable, the result of not getting enough rest and food. |
| 3.  **Child like mannerisms.** Similar to those displayed by much younger children such as thumb sucking, soiling of pants, temper tantrums. |
| 4.  **Fear of adults.** The child may start clinging to an adult for emotional support and may be quite fearful of adults. |
| 5. |
| 6.  **Very low self-esteem.**  Very low self esteem and may start having problems at school. |
| 7.  **Dirty clothing and unpleasant body odor.** Lack of basic health care such as dental work, glasses, hearing aid. |
| 8.  **Extreme behavior/aggressiveness.**  May show extreme behavior such as aggressiveness, destructive, hyperactive or shyness, or may not display any emotion at all. |
| 9. |
| 10.  **Reluctance to go home.**  May be reluctant to leave day care center or school. |
| To summarize, judge the following signs or indicators of child abuse. Observe carefully and asses the situations: |
|     ▪ Sleep disturbance (nightmares, fear of going to bed) |
|     ▪ Loss of appetite |
|     ▪ Behavior change (irritable, aggressiveness, withdrawn) |
|     ▪ Bed-wetting |
|     ▪ Clinging |
|     ▪ Fear of adults |
|     ▪ Not wanting to go home |
|     ▪ Regression |
|     ▪ Depression |

# 4.7         INFANT CARE

## 4.7.1   FEEDING

***In feeding a baby with milk...***

1. Tilt the bottle sufficiently so that the neck and tip are always full of milk. Too much air will be taken in by the baby if this is not allowed.
2. Remove the bottle occasionally during feeding to let the baby rest.
3. Let the baby burp after feeding or occasionally during feeding to remove air taken in by the baby.
4. To burp the baby, hold him over your shoulder and gently pat shoulder.
5. Dispose of left over milk after feeding since it can be contaminated with germs easily.

***In introducing or giving
home made food to the baby...***

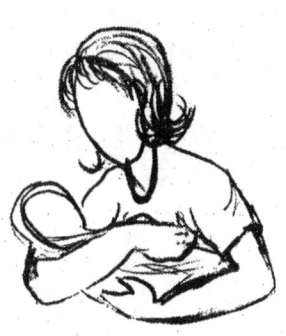

1. Avoid too much salt, sugar or any other spices as they can be harmful.
2. Make sure that all utensils to be used are thoroughly cleaned.
3. Avoid canned food products not especially prepared for babies. Fresh fruits and vegetables are preferred.

### *PREPARING MILK FEED*

Prior to the preparation of milk feed, be sure that bottles, teats, funnel and screw rings are thoroughly washed and sterilized to avoid contamination with infection causing bacteria.

***Steps in milk feed preparation...***

1. Wash hands thoroughly with clear water and soap before preparing the milk feed.
2. Bring to heat a large clean pan of drinking water.

3    While the water is heating, wash all feeding accessories with detergent soap and bottle brush. Rinse all utensils in cold water until completely free of soapy water.

4    Submerge all feeding accessories in the water being heated, cover the pan and boil for at least 10 minutes.

5    After 10 minutes, remove all utensils with a pair of clean tongs or a clean fork and put them on a clean fork and put them on a clean surface to drain. Pour away the remaining water. Bottles should be placed upside down.

6    Boil an appropriate amount of clean drinking water in a pan or bottle for about 5 minutes.

7    Pour the boiled water into the bottle and allow to cool to approximately 50%.

8    Add the correct amount of milk formula according to the feeding table or the doctor's advice. Use only the measuring scoop which is provided.

9    Close the feeding bottle with a clean cap and shake until the powder has dissolved completely.

10   Place the teat on the table without touching the part that goes into the baby's mouth. Allow to cook drinking temperature (approximately $35^0$ C - $37^0$ C)

## 4.7.2   BATHING A BABY

*Steps in bathing a baby...*

1    Give the baby his bath in his room, the kitchen or the bathroom before feeding.

2    Put a portable bath tub on the table or place a rectangular plastic dish pan in the kitchen sink.

3    Fill tub with warm water. See to it that the room temperature is at $21^0$ C.

4    Undress the baby quickly and place him at once in the warm water.

5    Thoroughly and gently wash the baby's body with a soft wash cloth rubbed with

mild soap while supporting the baby's head with one hand.

6    Wrap the baby loosely with a large bath towel when removing from the bath tub and place him in a small blanket.

7    Dress the baby quickly while he is held within the folds of the blanket.


## 4.7.3  DIAPERING – DRESSING A BABY

Dressing a baby is fairly difficult task because he normally turns, twists and rolls over. One must provide some sort of distraction with a favorite toy or musical box or by singing a song.


***Steps in Diapering
(dressing a baby)...***

1    The first and the old-fashioned way:
   a.)    Fold the diaper into a triangle with two inches thickness or more.
   b.)    The triangle is put under the buttocks with the two upper points brought across his abdomen and the third point between his legs and pinned onto the crossed points.

2    The second way or method:
   a.)    The diaper is folded into an oblong shape, the shorter sides of which are comfortably fit together around the baby's abdomen, and the diaper passes between his legs, and is pinned on both sides.

3    The third method:
   a.)    This is used for T-shaped diapers. The arms of the T is brought between the legs and pinned neatly at each side.

It must be emphasized that the diaper must not be tightly fitted to the baby's abdomen or between his legs, whatever method is used.

These interesting, easy to learn nursery rhymes are a delight treat for children. Learn them, teach them, act them out and say them often and let the wonderful world of songs and poems help you in stimulating the social, physical, intellectual, creative and emotional developmental of children.

## *CONTENTS*

# NURSERY RHYMES/POEMS

*These short nursery poems will delight the children under your care. They are also available in cassette tapes. It is a good enunciation lessons for caregivers whose mother tongue is not English. Instead of a native English speaker, I have decided to record them myself to serve as your model in acquiring English diction and intonation. Good Luck!*

[Proceeds from the sale of the tapes are used in producing more ESL resource materials]

*julie v. krachy*

### 1. ALL WORK AND NO PLAY

All work and no play
Makes one a dull boy;
All play and no work
Make one a mere toy.

### 2. ANIMAL FAIR4

I went to the animal fair
The birds and the beast were there,
The big babbon
By the light of the moon
Was combing his auburn hair
The monkey, he got drunk,
And sat on the elephant's trunk
The elephant sneezed,
And fell on his knees.

### 3. AS I WAS GOING TO SELL MY EGGS

As I was going to sell my eggs,
I met a man with bandy legs,
Bandy legs and crooked toes,
I tripped up his heels
And fell on his nose.

### 4. BAA, BAA, BLACK SHEEP

Baa, baa, black sheep,
Have you any wool?
Yes sir, yes sir,
Three bags full.
One for my master,
And one for my dame,
And one for the little boy,
Who lives down the lane.

### 5. FISHY, FISHY IN THE BROOK

Fishy, fishy in the brook
Daddy caught him with a hook;
Mommy fried in a pan
And baby ate him like a man!

### 6. HEY DIDDLE DIDDLE

Hey diddle diddle
The cat and the fiddle,
The cow jumped over the moon;
The little dog laughed
To see such sport,
And the dish ran away with the spoon.

### 7. HICKORY, DICKORY, DOCK

Hickory, dickory, dock
The mouse ran up the clock;
The clock struck one,
The mouse ran down,
Hickory, dickory, dock.

### 8. HIGGLETY, PIGGLETY, POP

Higglety, pigglety, pop!
The dog has eaten the mop;
The pig's in a hurry
The cat's in a flurry

Higglety, pigglety pop

And what became on the monk

The monk, the monk, a-choo!

### 9. HOW MANY DAYS

How many days has my baby to play?
Sunday, Monday, Tuesday, Wednesday,
Thursday, Friday, Saturday.
Hop away, skip away;
My baby wants to play,
My baby wants to play everyday!

### 10. HUMPTY DUMPTY

Humpty Dumpty sat on a wall,
Humpty Dumpty had a great fall.
All the king's horses,
And all the king's men
Couldn't put Humpty Dumpty togather again

### 11. HUSH-A-BYE, BABY

Hush-a-bye baby, on the tree top,
When the wind blows
The cradle will rock;
When the bough breaks
The cradle will fall,
Down will come baby, cradle and all.

### 12. I SEE THE MOON

I see the moon
And the moon sees me
God bless the moon
And God bless me.

### 13. JACK AND JILL

Jack and Jill went up the hill,
To fetch a full of water;
Jack fell down and broke his crown,
And Jill came tumbling after.

### 14. JACK BE NIMBLE

Jack be nimble,
Jack be quick
Jack jump over
The candlestick.

### 15. LITTLE DROPS OF WATER

Little drops of water,
Little grains of sand
Make a mighty ocean,
And the pleasant land.

And the little minutes
Humble though they may be,
Make the mighty ages
Of eternity.

### 16. MISTRESS MARY

Mistress Mary, quite contrary,
How does your garden and grow?
With cockle-shells, and silver bells,
And pretty maids all in a row

### 17. MIX A PANCAKE

Mix a pancake
Stir a pancake
Pop it in a pan;

Fry a pancake
Toss a pancake
Catch it if you can.

### 18. ONE THING AT A TIME

So work while you work
And play while you play
This is the way
To be happy and gay.

### 19. ONE, TWO BUCKLE MY SHOE

| | |
|---|---|
| One two | Buckle my shoe |
| Three, Four | Knock at the door |
| Five, six | Pick up sticks |
| Seven, eight | Lay them straight |
| Nine, ten | A big fat hen. |

### 20. ONE, TWO, THREE, FOUR, FIVE

One, two, three, four, five
I caught a fish alive;
Six, seven, eight, nine, ten!
I let her go again.

### 21. PAT-A-CAKE

Pat-a-cake, pat-a-cake
Baker's man
Bake me a cake
As fast as you can.
Pat it and prick it,
And mark it with a B
And put it in the oven
For baby and me.

### 22. RAIN, RAIN, GO AWAY

Rain, rain, go away
Come another day
Little Johnny wants to play.

### 23. RING-A-RING OF ROSES

Ring-a-ring of roses,
A pocket full of posies,
A-tishoo! A-tishoo!
We all fall down.

### 24. ROCK-A-BYE BABY

Rock a bye baby
On the tree tops,
When the wind blows
The cradle will rock;
When the bough breaks
The cradle will fall,
Down will come baby
Cradle and all.

### 25. ROSES ARE RED

Roses are red
Violets are blue
Sugar is sweet
And so are you

### 26. SEVEN BLACKBIRDS IN A TREE

Seven blackbirds in a tree,
Count them and see what they can be.
One for sorrow,
Two for joy,
Three for girl,
Four for boy,
Five for silver,
Six for gold,
Seven for secret,
That's never been told.

138

**27.  SING A SONG OF SIXPENCE**

Sing a song of sixpence
A pocket full of rye
Four and twenty blackbirds,
Baked in a pie.

When the pie was opened,
The birds began to sing;
Was not that a dainty dish,
To set before a king?

**28.  SING, SING, WHAT SHALL I SING?**

Sing, sing, What shall I sing?
The cat's run away
With the pudding string!
Do, Do, what shall I sing?
The cat has bitten it
Quite in two!

**29.  SLIDING**

Down the slide we ride, we ride.
Round we run and then
Up we pop to reach the top
And down we come again

**30.  THANK YOU GOD!**

Thank you  for the world so sweet,
Thank you for the food we eat,
Thank you for the birds that sing
Thank you God for everything.

**31.  THE OWL**

Of all the queer birds I ever did see,
The owl is the queerest by far to me.
For all the day long she sits in a tree,
And when the night comes away flies she!

**32.  THERE WAS A CROOKED MAN**

There was a crooked man,
And he went a crooked mile
He found a crooked sixpence,
Against a crooked stile;
Which brought a crooked mouse
And they all lived together
In a little crooked house!

**33.  THERE WAS AN OLD WOMAN**

There was an old woman
Who lived in a shoe
She had so many children
She didn't know what to do;
She gave them some brain
Without any bread;
She whipped them all soundly
And put them to bed.

**34.  THIS LITTLE PIG**

This little pig went to market,
This little pig stayed home,
This little pig had a roast beef,
This little pig had none,
And this little pig cried,
Wee-wee-wee-wee-wee
All the way home.

**35.  THIS LITTLE TURTLE**

There was a little turtle,
He lived in a box.
warm in a puddle,

He climbed on the rocks.
He snapped at a mosquito,
He snapped at fleas,
He snapped at a minnow.
And he snapped at me
He caught the mosquito
He caught the flea
He caught the minnow
But he didn't catch me.

**36.  THREE BLIND MICE**

Three blind mice, see how they run!
They all ran after the farmer's wife.
Who cut off their tails with a carving knife,
Did you ever see such a thing in your life,
As the three blind mice.

**37.  TOMMY TUCKER**

Little Tommy Tucker
Sings for his supper.
What shall he eat?
White bread and butter.
How shall he cut it
Without a knife?
How shall he marry
  Without a wife?

**38.  TRAFFIC LIGHT SONG**

I like to cross streets at the corner
Where the traffic signals glow.
The light at the top
Is red for "STOP"
The bottom one's green for "GO"
I look to the left
I look to the right'
I wait till its safe to go.
I like to cross streets at the corner
Where the traffic signals glow.

**39.  TWINKLE, TWINKLE LITTLE STAR**

Twinkle, twinkle little star
How I wonder what you are!
Up above the world so high,
Like a diamond in the sky,
Twinkle, twinkle little star,
How I wonder what you are!

## *CONTENTS*

**GAMES**

Below are the examples of games you and the children can play. Also visit the library with the child(ren) and take out book son games and things to do. In addition to acquiring the health habit of using the library as a resource for materials and ideas, taking field trips once a week or once every two weeks is an enriching activity that satisfies the social, physical, intellectual, creative, and emotional needs and activities of the children under your care.

| 1 |
| :---: |
| **BEETLE** |

***Rules:***
1 – Nose and mouth
2 – Eyes
3 – Feet and hands
4 – Arms and legs
5 – Head
6 – Body

6 members are needed to start the game. You need one die, paper and a pencil for each player (any number of players).

Each player throws the die and the first to throw a six starts the game.

Then, each player in turn throws the die, and draws the part of a beetle which his die number allows. Go on throwing in turn until one player has drawn a whole beetle. He is the WINNER!

| 2 |
| :---: |
| **BABY BASKETBALL** |

The purpose of this game is to develop large muscle coordination, and to give some background experience in a basic game.

There are many variations on this game. The equipment can range from a wicker clothes hamper, wastebasket, or playhouse window, to an actual child sized basketball game (Fischer – Price makes an excellent one). If you improvise the "basket", you'll also need small balls, bean bags, or blocks for the "ball"

Set up your "basket" a few feet away from the seated baby.

***Procedure:***
1. Getting down on the baby's level, crawl over to the basket and drop the ball into it. Repeat, saying, "Look, Kate! I made a basket!"
2. Hand a ball to the baby, saying. "Can Kate make a basket? Go on, drop it in!" if she reluctant to do so, encourage her by walking her over to the basket.
3. Take your turn again and then let your baby try it again. Sometimes a baby will sit watching intently but make no move to join in. continue to demonstrate a few more times. More than likely as soon as you leave her alone she'll creep over and try her luck.

## 3
## BELT HANGER

flat surface wooden coat hanger
cup hooks (6)
ribbon
enamel paint
ruler

1. Paint the wooden part of the hanger. Allow it to dry.
2. Next, measure off 6 places on the flat side of the hanger by making 3 pencil dots on either side of the hanger hook, an equal distance apart.
3. Lay the hanger flat, and screw the 6-cup hooks, evenly spaced, into the dots. (You may find it  easier to screw in the cup hooks if you make a small starter hole first, this can be done by pounding a small nail, such as flat head nail, a little way into the wood).
4. You can wind the hanger hook with ribbon or tie it with a perky bow.

## 4
## CHARADES

This is an excellent game for family parties, because most grown-ups enjoy it as much as children do. You don't even have to dress up, but it's more fun if you do, so it's a good idea to have a selection of odd hats, coats, scarves, sheets, dressing gowns, etc., all together in the room where you make your plans. Sometimes the clothes will suggest a word. But, in case you are all too excited to think clearly, it is a good idea to have a list of words to fall back on. Two-syllable words are enough for younger players. Here are some words, which work well and are easy to act: carrot, bargain, earwig, kidnap, partridge, knapsack, bandage and carpet. It will make the charade more difficult if you choose two words and act them both at the same time in order to confuse the audience.

| 5 CHRISTMAS TREE PRETTIES | |
|---|---|

4 cups flour      tempera paints      clear plastic spray
1 cup salt      paper clips
1 ½ cups water      thread

Note: As this involves using the oven, have an adult light it and set it for 350°F.
1. Mix the flour, salt and water to make a flour clay. Rub your hands with flour and knead the mixture for at least 5 minutes. At first the clay will be thin and sticky. Keep working it with your hands – it will thicken.
2. Next, mould the clay. You can shape Christmas wreaths, trees, stars or whatever strikes your fancy. For adding details, try using a toothpick to "etch" the clay. Finished pieces should be no thicker than ½ inch and no bigger than 3 inches.
3. Stick one end of a paper clip into each shape for a hook.
4. Cover a cookie sheet with foil and place your clay shapes on it. Bake in an oven at 350°F for about 12 – 20 minutes. When done, your clay will be a light brown color. When tapped with a fork, it will make a solid ringing sound.
5. Decorate your clay ornaments with paints. When paint is dry, spray ornaments with clear plastic coating. Tie a thread through each paper clip and trim a merry tree for the holidays.

| 6 FLOWER POT | |
|---|---|

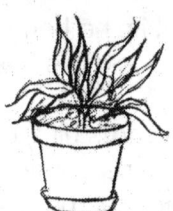

16 ounce coffee can (used)
tape measure
brightly colored, plastic cloth or contact paper
strong white glue
scissors

1. Rinse and dry the can. Using a nail, pound three (small) holes in the bottom.
2. Measure the height of the can from rim to rim and write down. Now measure the distance around the can, add an extra ½ inch for overlap, and write down that measurement also. Now mark your material and cut out the piece you will use.
3. Spread the "wrong" side of the piece with glue, especially along the edges, if not using contact paper. Put down one edge of the sticky side along the seam of the can and pull the piece firmly around the can until it overlaps. Press it down with your hands along sides and seam.
4. Pour enough pebbles into the can to cover the bottom, then fill halfway with soil.
5. Hold your plant so that the roots rest gently on this soil, then sift more soil to within one inch of the top. Press soil down gently and water. Set your potted plant on a saucer. WATCH IT GROW!

The purpose of this game is to enjoy some good rough and tumble fun. For this game, you need a third player, preferably a child between two and five years. The adult player is on all fours, with her back legs straddled and her backs straight, thus forming a tunnel or bridge for the baby to play on or under.

**Procedure:**
1. Introduce the game by calling to the older child to crawl under the bridge. Tell her to weave in and out between your arms and legs, too.
2. Call to the baby to follow the older child- "Come on, Kate, follow Amy!"
3. Tell the older child she can crawl up onto the top of the bridge (adult's back). Amy then slither, wriggling, down the other side, shouting, "Human jungle gym!"
4. Meanwhile, the baby continues to crawl under the bridge.
5. Teach the older child to call out, "Look out below!" and be careful not to land on the baby!

This game can be as rough as you want to make it for the older child, keeping in mind not to frighten the baby. A great game for a rainy day!

**7**
**H U M A N**
**J U N G L E**

**8**
**L E A P   F R O G**

Leap Frog is best played where it is soft to fall.

The first player makes a "back", that is, he bends well forward, holds with his hands, and tucks his head in.

Another player then makes a short run towards him, places his hands on his back and, with legs wide apart, leaps over him. He runs a few meters father ahead, and bends over to make another "back'. Any number of players can join in, each making a "back" after he has jumped over all the others.

Anyone who does not jump right over is out after three tries. The "backs" must stand very firma and the jumper should only rest his hands lightly on them.

| 9 | | |
|---|---|---|
| **PENCIL HOLDER** | | |

- 1 – 6 ¾ ounce frozen juice can (used)
- wool fabric or other heavy material
- yarn in a contrasting color
- darning needles
- glue
- scissors
- tape measure

1. Wash the juice can well and dry.
2. Measure the height and the distance around the can and use these measurements to cut out a piece of wool material to fit the can, allowing an extra ½ inch for overlap.
3. Using yarn, sew a blanket stitch along the top and bottom edges of your material. You can also embroider a flower design in the center of it.

Now smear the can with glue and press the piece of material firmly around the juice can.

The stitched borders should be at the top and bottom of your pencil holder. Let dry and use.

| 10 | |
|---|---|
| **SEVENS** | |

The idea is to throw the ball against the wall seven times, in seven different ways, and to catch it each time.

You need a rubber ball or tennis ball, a wall, and flat dry ground where the ball will bounce evenly.

1. Throw it directly onto the wall and catch it without it bouncing – seven times.
2. Throw it and let it bounce once and catch it seven-times.
3. Throw it and catch it with your right hand - seven times.
4. Throw it and catch it with your left hand – seven times.
5. Raise your right leg and with your right hand throw it under your leg and up to the wall and catch it –seven times.
6. Do the same procedure with the left leg and hand – seven times.
7. With your right hand, throw the ball around your back and up to the wall and catch it – seven times

There are lots of other ways and you can make some up yourself. But if you fail to catch a ball, you have to do that particular way all over again.

## 11
## SPONGE TOYS

- Graph paper
- Several colored sponges
- Waterproof glue
- Scissors

1. Trace outline of the sponge onto graph paper.
2. Now drawn a pattern that you desire and transfer it to the sponge shape you've drawn on the graph paper
3. Cut out the shape, pin it onto the sponge and cut out your sponge animal with sharp scissors.
4. Use the scraps from each sponge to make eyes, nose, mouth, etc., on the other animals. Glue these features on. Result: soft, waterproof toys for young children.

## 12
## SPLISH, SPLASH

- Sand bucket or unbreakable bowl
- Serving spoons
- Measuring cups or sand shovels

The purpose of this game is to have some good cool fun. First, find a good spot outdoors for the baby to play Splish, Splash. Place your baby in front of a half filled bucket of water. Get the baby started by gently splashing her hands in the water. If she enjoys it, give her a spoon or measuring cup to dip and splash with.

## 3
## THE FARMER'S IN HIS DEN

This can be played indoors and outdoors by boys and girls. The children makes a circle around one child, "the Farmer", who stands in the middle. The circle join hands and walk around the Farmer, singing:

**The Farmer's in his den,
the Farmer's in his den
Heigh-ho, heigh-ho,
the Farmer's in his den
The Farmer wants a wife,
the Farmer wants a wife
Heigh-ho, heigh-ho,
the Farmer wants a wife**

The circle stops and the Farmer chooses one child from the circle to be his "wife" and she joins him in the centre, the circle join hands again and walk around the Farmer and his wife, singing:

**The Wife wants a child,
the Wife wants a child
Height-ho, heigh-ho,
the Wife wants a child**

The Wife now chooses someone from the circle to be her child. The game goes on in the same way with everyone signing this verse:

**The Child wants a dog
The Child wants a dog
Heigh-ho, heigh-ho,
The Child wants a dog**

Then finally sing:

**We all pat the Dog
We all pat the Dog
Heigh-ho, heigh-ho
We all pat the Dog**

Everyone then pats the Dog, who is the Farmer next time if you play the game again.

# 4.10 CHILDREN'S STORIES

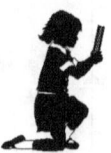

*To familiarize caregivers with classic stories children love to hear and learn, the following were summarized. Buy books that are colorful and easy to read and understand. Use the library as a resource area. Practice reading these stories aloud, they will exercise your tongue in expressing yourself aloud.*

**julie v. kallal**

## CONTENTS

1. Chicken Licken
2. Cinderella
3. Goldilocks & The Three Bears
4. Sleeping Beauty
5. The Little Red Hen
6. The Three Bily Goat Gruffs
7. The Three Little Pigs
8. The Wizard Of Oz

# 1.    Chicken Licken

*O*nce upon a time, there lived Chicken Licken. One day, while scratching in her garden, an acorn fell on her head.  She looked up and said "Oh, my, the sky is falling.  I better go and tell the King".

On her way to the King, she met Henny Penny. "Good morning, Chicken Licken, where are you going?"

"Oh Henny Penny, the sky is falling and I'm on my way to tell the King", said Chicken Licken.

"How do you know the sky is falling?" asked Henny Penny.

Chicken Licken said, "I saw it with my own two eyes, I heard it with my own two ears and a piece of it fell on my head!"

"Then I'll go with you", said Henny Penny.

So they went along until they met Cocky Locky. "Good morning Henny Penny and Chicken Licken, where are you going?", asked Cocky Locky.

"Oh Cocky Locky, the sky is falling and we are going t tell the King", answered Henny Penny.

"How do you know the sky is falling?", asked Cocky Locky.

"Chicken Licken told me" said Henny Penny.

"I saw it with my own two eyes, I heard it with my own two ears and a piece of it fell on my head!", said Chicken Licken.

"Then I'll go with you !", said Cocky Locky as he joined Henny Penny and Chicken Licken to tell the King that the sky is falling.

"Good morning, Cocky Locky, Henny Penny and Chicken Licken, where are you going?, said Ducky Duddles.

"Oh, Ducky Duddles, the sky is falling and we are going to tell the King!", answered Cocky Locky.

"How do you know the sky is falling?", asked Ducky Duddles.

"Henny Penny told me!", said Cocky Locky.

"Chicken Licken told me!", said Henny Penny.

"I saw it with my own two eyes, I heard it with my own two ears and a piece of it fell on my head!", said Chicken Licken.

"Then I'll go with you !", said Ducky Duddles as he joined Henny Penny and Chicken Licken to tell the King that the sky is falling.

"Good morning, Ducky Duddles, Cocky Locky, Henny Penny and Chicken Licken, where are you going?, said Goosey Loosey.

"Oh, Goosey Loosey, the sky is falling and we are going to tell the King!", answered Ducky Duddles.

"How do you know the sky is falling?", asked Goosey Loosey.
"Cocky Locky tole me!", said Dicky Duddles.
"Henny Penny told me!", said Cocky Locky.
"Chicken Licken told me!", said Henny Penny.

"I saw it with my own two eyes, I heard it with my own two ears and a piece of it fell on my head!", said Chicken Licken.

"Then I'll go with you !", said Goosey Loosey as he joined Ducky Duddles, Henny Penny and Chicken Licken to tell the King that the sky is falling.

"Good morning, Goosey Loosey, Ducky Duddles, Cocky Locky, Henny Penny and Chicken Licken, where are you going?, said Turkey Lurkey.

"Oh, Turkey Lurkey, the sky is falling and we are going to tell the King!", answered Goosey Loosey

"How do you know the sky is falling?", asked Turkey Lurkey.

"Ducky Lurky told me!", said Goosey Loosey.
"Cocky Locky tole me!", said Ducky Duddles.
"Henny Penny told me!", said Cocky Locky.

"Chicken Licken told me!", said Henny Penny. "I saw it with my own two eyes, I heard it with my own two ears and a piece of it fell on my head!", said Chicken Licken.

"Then I'll go with you !", said Turkey Lurkey as he joined Goosey Loosey, Ducky Duddles, Henny Penny and Chicken Licken to tell the King that the sky is falling.

Then they met Foxy Woxy. "Good morning, Turkey Lurkey, Goosey Loosey, Ducky Duddles, Cocky Locky, Henny Penny and Chicken Licken, where are you going?, said Foxy Woxy.

"Oh, Foxy Woxy, the sky is falling and we are going to tell the King!", answered Turkey Lurkey.

"How do you know the sky is falling?", asked Foxy Woxy.

"Chicken saw it with her own two eyes, she heard it with her own two ears and a piece of it fell on her head!", chorused Turkey Lurkey, Goosey Loosey, Ducky Duddles, Cocky Locky and Henny Penny.

"Yes, that's true and now we are on our way to tell the King!, said Chicken Licken.

"Then we will run and use a short cut near my den, so that we can tell the King that the sky is falling!",

So they all ran and use a short cut near his den, and the King was never told that the sky is falling.

And Foxy Woxy lived  happily ever after.


## 2.      Cinderella


$O$nce upon a time, there lived a beautiful, young girl. Her name was Cinderella. She lived with stepmother and two stepsisters. They treated her as a maid. She worked very hard. She worked all day and only when evening came was she allowed to rest. She liked resting near the fire, near the cinders. That was how she got her nickname, Cinderella.

Cinderella was in rags, while her stepsisters wore elegant clothes. But in spite of all this, Cinderella was beautiful while her stepsisters were ugly and had bad manners.

One day, they all learned that there was to be a ball at the palace. Cinderella wanted to go but her stepmother would not let her. Instead, she helped her stepsisters dress. She ironed their gowns, fetched water for their baths and polished their shoes. Cinderella was so broken hearted because she wanted to go, but even she wanted, she did not have a gown to wear and she looked so shabby.

When everybody was gone and Cinderella was resting near the fire, a burst of light appeared and a lovely fairy appeared before her.

"I'm your fairy godmother. I'll change you so you can go to the ball. You'll be the loveliest guest and the prince will notice you. But remember, you must leave by midnight! Now get me a pumpkin and tell your mice friends to come".

The fairy turned Cinderella into a beautiful lady, the pumpkin into a sparkling coach and six of the mice, she turned into six white horses and the seventh into a coachman. Cinderella could not believe her eyes and she was so happy

When Cinderella entered the ballroom at the palace, a hush fell. Everyone stopped to ask who she was and admired her beauty, charm and grace

The Prince noticed her at once. He approached her, bowed deeply and asked her to dance. In fact, from then on, he only danced with Cinderella all evening. Cinderella's stepsisters were so jealous and angry but they did not know that the Prince was dancing with their stepsister, Cinderella.

Time went by and all of a sudden, the clock started to strike. "Midnight", gasped Cinderella, "I must leave at once". And she ran all across the ballroom and down the long stairway where she lost one of her slippers. But she had no time to stop and pick it up. If the last stroke of midnight were to sound . . . she would be in big trouble! She fled from the palace and into the darkness of the night.

The Prince trying to run after her, saw her slipper. He picked it up. He summoned his soldiers to take the slipper into town the following day and to come back with its owner. His mind was made up. He would make the owner of the slipper his queen.

So the soldiers went all over town, and fit every girl in town with the slipper, but no one could fit into it. Soon, they came to Cinderella's house. The two stepsisters struggled in vain to fit their big feet into the little slipper. The soldiers gave up and were about to go when they noticed Cinderella in a corner. The Stepsisters and stepmother laughed for they were very certain that Cinderella's foot would not fit into the slipper.

Cinderella tried it on. It was a perfect fit. At that moment, the fairy appeared and raised her magic wand. And Cinderella's dress was transformed again into an elegant dress. Cinderella's stepmother and stepsisters gasped at her in amazement while her friends, the cat, the birds and the mice were singing with joy.

The soldiers took Cinderella and presented her to the prince. The queen was found at last. The whole kingdom rejoiced when the prince announce his wedding. The Prince and Cinderella lived happily ever after.

## 3.    Goldilocks & The Three Bears

Once upon a time, there lived three bears, Papa Bear, Mama Bear and Tiny Wee Bear.

One day, while waiting for their porridge to cool off, they decided to go for a walk in the woods.

While they were gone, along came a young little girl with beautiful golden locks. Her name was Goldilocks. She saw the house in the woods while gathering some flowers and decided to visit it. But no one was home.

The door to the kitchen was not locked, so she came in, saw three bowls of porridge on the table. She tasted the porridge in the great big bowl, but it was way too hot. She tasted the porridge in the middle-sized bowl, but it was still too hot. So she tasted the porridge in the tiny wee bowl and ate it all up.

Then she went into the living room and found three chairs. She tries to sit in Papa Bear's chair but it was way too hard. Then she tried Mama Bear's chair, but it was too soft. So she tried Tiny Wee Bear's chair and it was just right for her. So she sat right in but the chair broke.

By this time, Goldilocks was starting to get tired. So she went upstairs and saw three beds. She tried Pap Bear's bed but it was too big. She tried Mama Bear's bed but it was still big for her. So she tried Tiny Wee Bear's bed and it was just  right. So she jumped right in, covered herself and went fast asleep.

Soon the three bears came. In the kitchen Papa Bear said in a great big voice. "Somebody has been tasting my porridge!" Mama Bear looked into her bowl and said in her middle-sized voice, "Somebody has been tasting my porridge!" Tiny Wee Bear looked into her empty tiny wee bowl and cried, "Somebody has been tasting my porridge and has eaten it all up.

So they went to the living room and Papa Bear said in a great big voice. "Somebody has been sitting in my chair!" Mama Bear looked said in her middle-sized voice, "Somebody has been sitting in my chair!" And Tiny Wee Bear cried, "Somebody has been sitting in my chair and has broken it all to pieces.

Then they climbed into their bedroom. Papa Bear growled. "Somebody has been lying in my bed!" Mama Bear exclaimed, "Somebody has been lying in my bed!" And Tiny Wee Bear pointed, "Look! Somebody has been lying in my bed and here she is!"

At the moment, Goldilocks woke up, saw the three bears, go out of the bed and jumped out of the nearest window into the woods. The three bears never saw Goldilocks again and

Goldilocks never came to visit the three bears again. So Pap Bear, Mama Bear, Tiny Wee Bear and Goldilocks lived happily ever after.

## 4.    SLEEPING BEAUTY

*O*nce upon a time there lived a Queen who had a beautiful baby daughter. She invited all the fairies in the kingdom for the christening. Unfortunately, she missed one fairy who was a bit with as well. The fairy came anyway, but as she passed the baby's cradle, she whispered:

"When you turn sixteen, you will prick yourself with a spindle and die". One of the other fairies heard her and although, she could not entirely change the entire spell, chanted a magic spell to lighten the curse. "When you prick yourself, instead of dying, you would fall into a very deep sleep."

Years went by, the little princess grew into the most beautiful girl in the whole kingdom. Her mother was always very careful to keep her away from spindles. But on her sixteenth birthday, as she wandered through the castle, the princess came into a room where an old servant was spinning. And before the servant could stop her, the princess touched the spindle and pricked herself. She immediately dropped to the floor. The court doctors and the wizards were summoned, but there was nothing they could do. The fairies came too but they could not uncast the spell. One of them said however, that if love came along and a man of pure heart were to fall in love with her, that would bring her back to life.

The sleeping princess was taken to her room and laid on a bed of flowers. She was so beautiful and one of the fairies thought that it might take a hundred years before somebody came along and she could not let her princess wake up to strangers. So she cast another spell. Everyone who lived in the castle fell into a deep sleep. "When you wake up, lovely princess, those around you will wake up too!"

The years passed. The trees grew wild, the bushes became thick and straggly, the grass invaded the courtyards and the creepers spread the walls because nobody was awake to look after things. After a hundred years the castle was hidden in a dense forest.

One day, a young and handsome Prince wandering through the forest and saw the hidden castle. He explored the grounds and seeing that the drawbridge was down decided to cross over it and went into the castle. He saw the inhabitants draped all over, the stairs, the floors, the halls and even the courtyards. He thought they were all dead but realized that they were only asleep. He tried waking them up, but nobody moved. The Prince finally reached the room where the lovely Princess was sleeping. For a long time, he stood gazing at her face, so peaceful, so lovely, and pure. Suddenly, he felt the love he had always been searching for and never found, stirred his heart. Overcome by emotion, he came close, lifted the Princess dainty hand and planted a kiss.

At that kiss, the Princess opened her eyes. The spell was broken. The Princess and the whole castle became alive again. The Prince and Princess live happily ever after.

## 5.    THE WIZARD OF OZ

*O*nce upon a time, there lived a little girl named Dorothy. She had a dog named Toto and they both lived with Aunt Em and Uncle Henry.

One day, a whirlwind came while Aunt Em and Uncle Henry were away. It lifted the house where Dorothy and Toto were playing. It landed in the land of the Munchkins, on the top of the wicked witch of the East. The witch died. The Munchkins were happy because Dorothy and Toto saved them from the Wicked Witch. Dorothy and Toto wanted to go home but the Munchkins could not help them. But they gave her a pair of magic shoes that belonged to the wicked Witch of the East and told her to follow the yellow brick road to the Emerald City. "There you can ask the Wizard of Oz to help you", the Munchkins said.

So Dorothy and Toto started to skip along the yellow brick road." Suddenly, they met a Scarecrow. "Oh, Dorothy, I want to go with you to the wizard of Oz. I would like him to give me a brain". The Scarecrow hopped onto the yellow brick road and joined Dorothy and Toto.

Soon they met a Tin Man. "I have no heart and maybe the Wizard of Oz can help me. So, can I come with you?" asked the Tin Man, and along they all went.

Then they found a lion hiding behind a tree. "Please, Dorothy, take me with you so I can ask the Wizard of Oz for some courage!" Off they all went hopping along the yellow brick road.

Soon they reached the emerald City where everything was green. The Wizard of Oz lived in a palace. He asked the group what they wanted.

Dorothy said, "I would like to go home with my pet Toto, can you please help?" The scarecrow pleaded, "I would like to have a brain, can you please help?" The Tin Man squeaked, "I would like a heart, can you please help me?" the Lion roared, "I would like some courage, can you please help?"

The Wizard of Oz looked at each of the group and gave one determined answer. "I'll give you what you each want if you can chase the Wicked Witch of the West from the Emerald City." The group had no choice but to find the Wicked Witch of the West.

Everyone in Emerald City was afraid of the Wicked Witch of the West but not Dorothy. She came face to face with her and she and her group overpowered the Wicked Witch of the West and drove her out of the Emerald City.

The Wizard was so happy that he awarded the Scarecrow with a brain, the Tin Man with a heart, the Lion with some courage and Dorothy and Toto their way home. And they all lived happily ever after.

## 6. The Little Red Hen

Once upon a time, there lived Little Red Hen. One day, while scratching in a field, she found a grain of wheat. "Who will plant this grain of wheat?" she asked.

"Not I," said the Duck.
"Not I," said the Cat.
"Not I, "said the Dog.
"Then I will," said the Little Red Hen. And she did.

Soon, the wheat is ripe. "Who will harvest the wheat?" asked the Little Red Hen.

"Not I," said the Duck.
"Not I," said the Cat.
"Not I, "said the Dog.
"Then I will," said the Little Red Hen. And she did.

When the wheat was threshed, The Little Red Hen asked, "Who will take this wheat to the mill?"

"Not I," said the Duck.
"Not I," said the Cat.
"Not I, "said the Dog.
"Then I will," said the Little Red Hen. And she did.

She took the wheat tot the mill and had it ground on the floor. "Who will make this flour into bread?" the Little Red Hen asked.

"Not I," said the Duck.
"Not I," said the Cat.
"Not I, "said the Dog.
"Then I will," said the Little Red Hen. And she did.

She baked the bread. Then she asked, "Who will eat this bread?"

"I will!" said he Duck.
"I will!" said the Cat.
"I will!" said the Dog.
"Oh, no!" said the Little Red Hen. "I will eat the bread myself!" And she did.

## 7.    THE THREE BILLY GOATS GRUF

Once upon a time, there were three Billy Goats and they were all named Gruf.

One day, they decided to go up to the hillside to  make themselves fat.  They had to cross a bridge where a great ugly troll lived.

The youngest Bill Goat Gruf tried to cross the bridge first.

"Trip, trap, trip, trap," went the bridge.

"Who's that tripping over my bridge! I'm hungry and I'm going to gobble you up!, roared the Troll.

"It's only I, the tiniest and the thinnest Billy goat. I'm going to the other side to fatten me up. Wait
for a second Billy Goat; he's much bigger and fatter!", said the tinniest Billy Goat Gruf.

"Off with you then," said the Troll.

"Trip, trap, trip, trap," went the bridge.

"Who's that tripping over my bridge! I'm hungry and I'm going to gobble you up!, roared the Troll.

"Oh, don't bother with me! I'm going to the other side to fatten me up. Wait for my big brother; he's right behind me!", said the second Billy Goat Gruff.

"Very well, be off with you!," said the Troll.

"TRIP…TRAP..TRIP…TRAP moaned the bridge for the third Billy Goat Gruf was so heavy.

"Who's that tripping on my bridge? I'm not waiting any longer. I'm coming to eat you up!"

"Come along then!" the Billy Goat Gruff said and met the Troll on the bridge with his two great spears and tossed him back over the bridge and into the dirty water.

So the three Billy Goat Grufs fattened themselves up on the other side of the bridge and the Troll never bothered any one of them anymore, and they all lived happily ever after.

## 8. THE THREE LITTLE PIGS

Once upon a time there lived three little pigs and their mother.

One day, their mother decided to let her three pigs go and seek their own fate and fortunes.

The first little pig went away and soon met a man with a bundle of straw.  "Would you please give me your straw so I could build me a house?", the first little pig said.  The man gave the straw to the little pig.  The little pig lived in his house, which he built from straw.

Then the bad wolf came along and knocked at the door of the little straw house.  "Little pig, little pig, let me come in!", called the wolf.  "No, no, by the hair of my chinny chin chin, I'll not let you in!" , answered the little pig.  "Then I'll huff and I'll puff and I'll blow your house in", said the wolf.

So he huffed and he puffed and he blew the house in but the little pig got away.

The second little pig went away and soon met a man with a bundle of sticks.  "Would you please give me your sticks so I could build me a house?", the second little pig said.  The man gave the bundle of sticks and the little pig lived in his house which he built from sticks.

Soon the big bad wolf came along and knocked at the door of the house that was made of sticks.  "Little pig, little pig, let me come in!", called the wolf.  "No, no, by the hair of my chinny chin chin, I'll not let you in!" , answered the little pig.  "Then I'll huff and I'll puff and I'll blow your house in", said the wolf.

So he huffed and he puffed and he blew the house in and again the little pig that built the house made of sticks got away.

The third little pig  went away and soon met a man with a load of bricks.  "Would you please give me your load of bricks so I could build me a house?", the third little pig said. The man gave the bricks to the little pig and he built himself a brick house.

Soon the big bad wolf came to the door of the house that was made of bricks. "Little pig, little pig, let me come in!", called the wolf.
"No, no, by the hair of my chinny chin chin, I'll not let you in!" , answered the little pig. "Then I'll huff and I'll puff and I'll blow your house in", said the wolf. So he huffed and he puffed but he could not blow the little brick house in. Then he finally said, "If you won't let me in through the door, then I'll climb up on the roof and come down through the chimney", said the wolf. But the little pig made the fire in the chimney very hot and the wolf finally gave up and went away.

So the little pig went back to his mother to pick her up. He saw the other two pigs and invited them also to live with him. The three little pigs and their mother lived happily ever after.

## 4.11            QUESTIONS

1. What is the normal pulse rate of a newborn baby?

2. What is the normal respiratory rate of a new born baby and the characteristic of the baby's breathing?

3. What is the normal blood pressure of a baby at birth and after 10 days?

4. What is milia?

5. What is lanugo?

6. What do the following terms mean?
   **Blink Reflex:**
   **Rooting Reflex:**
   **Sucking Reflex:**
   **Extrusion Reflex:**
   **Tonick Neck Reflex**
   **Moro Reflex:**

7. What is colic and its causes?

8. How do you prevent colic?

9. What are the ages and stages of child development?

10. What are the psychosexual stages of the infant, toddler, preschooler and schooler according to Freud?

11. What are the psychosocial stages of the infant, toddler, preschooler and schooler according to Erickson?

12. What are the types of play for infant, toddler, preschooler and schooler?

13. What are the purposes of play?

14. What are the appropriate toys for the infant, toddler, preschooler and schooler?

15. What are the greatest fears of an infant, toddler, preschooler and schooler?

16. Differentiate growth and development.

17. Why does a child need to feel safe?

18. What are the basic development needs of children?

19. What are physical needs?

20. What are social needs?

21. What are intellectual needs?

22. What are creative needs?

23. What are emotional needs?

24. What will you do if the child is masturbating?

25. What will you do if the child asks about sex?

26. Why does a child have tantrums?

27. How do you manage temper tantrums?

28. How do you develop the speech of the child?

29. How do you develop the thinking and reasoning skills of a child?

30. What will you do if the child bites another child?

31. How do you encourage the independence of the child?

32. How do you help the child to feel special?

33. What is diaper rash?

34. How to avoid diaper rash?

35. At what age do you start to toilet train the child?

36. How do you know that a child is ready for toilet training?

37. At what age does a child eat his first solid food? What kinds of food should be prepared for a baby?

38. At what age does a child first learn to feed himself even with uncoordinated movements?

39. At what age does a child learn to use a spoon and a fork while eating?

40. Differentiate fine from gross motor skills.

41. How do you keep the child safe in the house?

42. What are the acceptable approaches in child management?

43. How do you burp a baby?

44. What is Down's Syndrome and its characteristics?

45. What is asthma and its signs and symptoms?

46. How is asthma attack prevented?

47. What will you do if the child is having an asthma attack?

48. What will you do if the child is suffering from toothache?

49. How do you handle fighting children?

50. What is autism?

51. How do you handle an autistic child?

How will you manage a child with poor appetite?

# MODULE
## 5A
### CARE FOR THE ELDERLY

MODULE OBJECTIVES

**By the end of the module, the participants will be able to:**

- Identify the three phases and types of aging.
- Describe the role of caregiver.
- Appreciate the rights of the elderly.
- Describe the needs and
activities of the elderly.
- Understand the relationship between aging and nutrition.
- Recognize illness and disabilities due to aging.
- Know how to care for an elderly with disabilities.
- Perform personal and basic nursing care for the elderly.
- Apply knowledge and skills gained during class sessions.

**MODULE 5**

MODULE 5

CARE OF THE SENIOR/Persons with Special Needs
TOTAL ALLOTED TIME - 120 HOURS

TERMINAL OBJECTIVES OF MODULE 5A

Upon completion of Module 5A, the participant will be able to:

♦ identify the three phases and types of aging
♦ describe the role of the caregiver
♦ appreciate the rights of the elderly
♦ understand the relationship between aging and nutrition
♦ recognize illness and disabilities due to aging
♦ know how to care for an elderly with disabilities
♦ perform personal and basic nursing care for the elderly
♦ apply knowledge and skills gained during class sessions

## MODULE 5A OUTLINE

| TOPICS | SUB-TOPICS TOTAL TIME - | LEARNING SITES/TIMES (Classroom) | | |
|---|---|---|---|---|
| | | Classroom & FILMS & Workbooks (114 hrs) | *One-on-One Assessment of Critical Skills 2 hrs | How to: 6 hours |
| 5.1 Three Phases of Aging | 5.1.1 The Pre-Retirement Phase 5.1.2 The Retirement Phase 5.1.3 The Post Retirement Phase | | | a. safe-proof the house b. wash hands and prevent germs from spreading c. feed a bedridden elderly |
| 5.2 Types of Aging | 5.2.1 Chronological Aging     6.2.3 Psychological Aging 5.2.2 Biological Aging          6.2.4 As a Companion | | | |
| 5.3 The Roles of the Caregiver | 5.3.1 As an Employee          6.3.3. As a Provider of Care 5.3.2 As a "Member" of the Family     6.3.4 As a Companion | | | d. exercise legs, hands, neck, body (deep breathing) |
| 5.4 Traits | 5.4.1 Case Studies Leading to the Identification of the Various          Characteristics of the Elderly Requiring Care | | | e.. effectively communicate |
| 5.5 Needs and Activities | 5.5.1 The Importance of a Checklist of Needs and Activities 5.5.2 General Care          6.5.3 Personal & Nursing Care | | | f. arrange social & outdoor activities g. arrange social visits to & from families & friends |
| 5.6 Aging and Nutrition | 5.6.1 Factors Affecting Nutrition 5.6.2 Food Groups & Nutrition | | | h. care for the feet |

| 5.7 Aging and Disabilities | 5.7.1 Aging & Disabilities | | | |
|---|---|---|---|---|

TEXT: THE CAREGIVER RESOURCE MANUAL

*Julie V. Kallal*

# CONTENTS OF MODULE 5A

5a.6.4 Common Illnesses And Diseases Of The Elderly (Glossary)

# 5A.1                PHASES OF AGING

Three distinct phases of aging:

**4-25**

### Pre-Retirement Phase

> This phase can begin as early as age 50, when individuals start to consciously wonder and think of life after adulthood.

### Retirement Phase

- At age 65, the onset of the second phase of aging, an aging adult experiences a temporary crisis in life. His 65th birthday can precipitate many doubts and adjustments. He has now retired from work.
- Depending on how prepared he is for his retirement, a person can welcome this second phase with enthusiasm and continue to be very productive and active.
- Health, financial stability, and lifestyle are major factors in influencing the quality of life at this stage.

### Post-Retirement Phase

- This third phase may also be referred to as the "Senility Phase". It is characterized by the aging person exhibiting many of the diseases and disabilities associated with aging.
- Seniors going into this phase are likely to have more medical problems as well as physical complaints.
- The sections on the Care for the Elderly address this third phase specifically. Bear in mind that many seniors especially those who have meticulously planned for their retirement may not experience many of the adjustment problems that are mentioned in this text.

Although the three phases seem to be distinct, well-defined and different, the problem facing the family of the elder or the elderly himself is when extra care is needed, or if it is needed at all. A trip to the doctor once in a while may no longer be enough and cannot always be provided by a family member anymore. A senior may not notice that he is now spilling food too often or can no longer dress himself without extra help. Maybe the most difficult is when a senior can no longer live by himself or in the case of husband and wife, may no longer be able to help each other and my now require outside help.

**Aging is a complex process which is universal, inevitable, and irreversible.**

## 5A.2         TYPES OF AGING

**Chronological**    Associated with the passage of time

**Biological**    Associated with the physical changes that occur with the passage of time

**Psychological**    Associated with the concept of self-worth with the passage of time.

**Social**    Associated with the relationship with families, friends and the community with the passage of time

## 5A.3    THE ROLE OF THE CAREGIVER FOR THE  ELDERLY

### What Every Caregiver MUST Perform:

| | | |
|---|---|---|
| 1 | **Know the elderly's characteristics and personality.** | Every caregiver must know a lot of things about the elderly such as likes, dislikes, family, ailments, etc. Only then will the caregiver be able to understand the needs and behavioral dynamics of the aging employer. |
| 2 | **Know and understand his/her other responsibilities, duties, and tasks.** | Every caregiver must be sensitive to the needs of the elderly and plans to satisfy those needs. |
| 3 | **Individualize and find answers to questions about the elderly.** | a. How is the bent, fragile, white haired lady with shaking hands different from her equally elderly friend who visits her from time to time?<br>b. What are the unique abilities, interests, problems, and strengths of each of these seniors that he/she encounters daily?<br>c. How varied, exciting, traumatic are each lifetime experience?<br>d. What is this senior's purpose in joining some senior groups?<br>e. What skills and personality strengths can the senior share with others?<br>f. What are the senior's weaknesses, ailments, chronic problems?<br>g. Has the senior accepted the consequences of aging? |
| 4 | **Express warmth and concern towards the welfare of the elderly.** | Especially to an elderly with a poor self-image and many feelings of inferiority, a caregiver must provide reassurance toward the senior's action, ignore negative behavior and have patience and stamina for change of moods. |
| 5 | **Give hope to the elderly.** | This is one of the most important skills in working with an elderly who has given up hope that life can ever be any better. Without hope, there can be no change. |
| 6 | **Assist as little as possible in tasks that the senior can usually handle him/herself.** | The less dependent the elderly is on you, the more independent he/she feels. |

| 7 | Use the elderly's wisdom and make him/her feel needed and wanted. | Be generous in your expressions of appreciation towards his/her advice and ideas. |
|---|---|---|
| 8 | Encourage elderly to socialize, to volunteer and to visit his/her family. | Do not stay too long during visits, the elderly is much more appreciated that way. |
| 9 | When friends and relatives neglect to call, remind them. | Remind relatives that a call once every two weeks is very much appreciated and really looked forward to by the elderly.  Remind them also that children's calls are equally important or that when calling, grandchildren can say a quick hello on the phone. |
| 10 | Be a good listener. | Many times, the elderly may simply want you to listen.  Avoid put downs and taking sides. |
| 11 | Smile a lot. | Be a friend and companion. |
| 12 | Learn how to keep secrets. | When an elderly is upset, he may speak his mind without due regard to who is listening.  Become a selective listener and avoid repeating matters that may not be welcomed by others. |
| 13 | Be updated on elderly's health condition. | As elderly's health deteriorates and more needs surface, find out how to cope with them and share your knowledge with others. |
| 14 | Maintain your self-composure and avoid stress. | Go over your coping mechanism sheet in order to maintain your composure and balance. |

## 5A.3.1 THE RIGHTS OF THE ELDERLY

### Self-Determination

The elderly has the right to decide and determine what is best.

### Personal Dignity.

The elderly has the right to his dignity and pride.

| | |
|---|---|
| **Privacy of Person and Thought.** | **Excellent Medical Care.** |
| The elderly's private body and thoughts should be respected. | The elderly has the right to a medically sound care. |
| **Personal Care.** | **Have Social Needs Met.** |
| The elderly has the right to be enjoyed by others in terms of his hygiene. | The elderly has the right to enjoy his family and friends. |

## 5A.3.2 THE CHARACTERISTICS OF THE ELDERLY

The following anecdotes describe the characteristics of the elderly and the process of getting old. Each anecdote describes some personality changes that evolve as individuals age.

**1**

**And it wasn't easy,** you know living alone. It was hard breaking up a home that you've had. And you know, I entertained a lot and had a lot of friends. They always felt free to come in. Well, of course, it's limited here. They never come any more. I miss the activities and the laughter. I don't seem to be able to do what I did before. I feel so alone in spite of my new friends here.

**2**

**No! No! I can bathe myself.** Just leave me alone. I can do it by myself. I did not want you here. I could manage by myself. I always have. You think I'm senile, huh! Don't touch me!

**3**

**That night the evening shift** was also short of help. There were four people to do the work of nine. The shortage was so great that even RNs on the shift were changing bedding for the patients. Early in the evening a senior caregiver was putting a patient to bed. The patient had soiled himself and his bed. According to the nurse, the caregiver had "the good sense" to change him and change his linen. He undressed the patient and helped him into the bathtub. While the patient was enjoying his bath, the caregiver went to get a towel and some clean linen. But there were none on the floor at that time. The janitor happened to be mopping the floor at the time so without thinking, the caregiver asked him if he could keep an eye while she went to get some fresh towels. When she returned she found the janitor helping the patient out of a tub full of scalding water. They wrapped him in a clean sheet and put him to bed. They did not tell the nurse what happened. About an hour after the patient was scalded, the evening the nurse came and "just happened" to look in on the patient. There, lying in bed, in a state of shock was the patient, with skin so red and blisters all over his body. The discovery was gruesome, an ambulance was called but the patient died after two weeks in the hospital.

## 4

**One 69 year old woman** was living with her son and daughter-in-law. The mother and daughter-in-law had never gotten along and couldn't tolerate talking to each other. The mother was discouraged from participating in any housework. She therefore would remain in her pajamas all day, watching television. When her son was due home, she would dress, put on her make-up and become warm and friendly. She and the daughter-in-law would compete for attention. The mother would complain that she was not invited to help the family and was considered a burden. The daughter-in-law would confirm that her mother-in-law was a burden. The son, caught in the middle, was forced to ask his mother to leave.

## 5

**The old man is dying** in the house. All the family is inside, the children too. The parents tell the children that they are going to say good-bye to the old man because they are never going to see him again. He is going to eternity. Some weep, one says to the person who is dying, "I am never going to see you again" and then cries. The neighbors visit also. "You are going to get well"; "You're not going to die"; "You're going to be healthy again". The children say "Many thanks for taking care of us. We'll miss you Grandpa". The old says farewell and sleeps, never to wake up again.

## 6

**An 80 year old man** was complaining to this friend. "My secretary is suing me for breach of promise." His friend answered, "At eighty five, what could you promise her?"

## 7

**The famous man from Yakuta**, who was found during the 1965 census to be 130 years old, received especially great publicity because he lived in a place with the most miserable climate with temperatures ranging from
-50°C to -60°C. When publicity about him became known world wide and a large article with picture of this outstanding man was published, a letter was received from a group of an ethnic villagers. Apparently, the villagers recognized this centenarian as a fellow villager who deserted from the army during the first world war and forged documents or used his father's identification (most usual method of falsification) to escape remobilization. It was found that this man was really only 99 years old.

## 8

**My society withdraws from me just as I withdraw from society. It is mutually agreed upon.**

## 9

**And now I am alone.** My husband has left me. I've repeatedly told him to go see the doctor but only I go. What am I going to do now?

**10**

**I am unable to chew.** My dentures no longer stay firm along my jaw. The nutritionist insists I eat meat for protein. Instead, I prefer mashed potatoes for it does not only fill me up, I don't even have to chew it. Fruits, what kind of fruits, they are hard and hard to chew. Processed fruits are expensive and my budget is limited. I'm not staying in this world for long anyway. It is best to save for my funeral.

**11**

**I am from primitive society.** Because I have grown stupid, old, wrinkled and weak, I am treated badly. My relatives took all my properties and now I don't have any. Recently, I have become unprotected and treated worse and worse. I am half-starved, hiding in corners, picking up bits and pieces of food from garbage bins.

**12**

**I am happy in my old age.** Of my wisdom, the young always respect. They listen and they seek for the many advices that I have ample to give. The fruits of my labor and the years of knowing are finally being recognized and sought for.

**13**

**Years and years of training and experience.** Now I don't remember. I would like to share and to give but I am too feeble to give. I can't even ask for a cup of coffee because I forget what to ask for.

**14**

**I tell you that a good relationship, ladies and gentlemen,** with your children, in your old age, depends to a large extent, on the graces and autonomy of the aged parent; in short, our ability to manage gracefully by ourselves. It would appear that in our own culture, there simply cannot be any happy role reversals between generations. There is neither an increasing dependency of parent upon child nor a continuing reliance of children upon parents. The parent must remain strong and independent. If his personal resources fail, then conflicts arise. The child on the other hand, must not threaten the security of the parent with request for monetary aid and other care when parental income has shrunk through retirement. The ideal situation is when both parent and child are functioning well. The parent does not depend on the child for nurturing or social interaction; these needs can be managed by the parent himself elsewhere. He does not limit the freedom of his child nor arouse the child's feeling of guilt. The child establishes an independent dwelling, sustains his own family, and achieves a measure of hope the parents had entertained for him. Such an ideal situation, of course, is more likely to occur when the parent is still provided with a spouse and where both the child and parents' socioeconomic status are preserved. In short, expect the worse of your situation. We, the aged, are at the mercy of time and society. Thank you.

**15**

**I am a widow.** I exist on a tiny allowance from my pension fund. My husband's serious illness and subsequent death wiped out our lifelong savings in just a few months. I have suffered chronic health problems for ten years, a residual effect of a serious illness from which I successfully recovered.

## 16

**I rely on friends and relatives** to take me to the doctor during my regular check-up because I don't drive and the bus terminal is five blocks from me. I feel so obligated and feel that my friends and relatives sometimes resent me.

## 17

**My post retirement activity** represents a relatively sharp change in the content of my experience. At the time of my full retirement, I was confronted by a series of invitations and opportunities to engage in continued professional work in various cities and far away as possible. On reflection, my wife and I decided to reject all of them. I had more than enough of riding in airplanes and living in hotels. We wished to stay here among our friends. This gives me the opportunity to activate a long, smoldering interest in painting. The painting now claims my primary interest and labor and I have become the president of our local art club. I keep some professional work going and this gives me a sense of achievement and a new kind of fulfillment.

## 5A.5       NEEDS AND ACTIVITIES OF THE ELDERLY

A checklist of needs and activities can identify quite simply the needs and activities of the elderly who require care. Initially, the checklist is done to assess and determine a baseline in which to outline the duties and responsibilities of the caregiver. Thereafter, the checklist is used to progressively identify and expand not only the developmental nature of the elder's needs and activities, but the caregiver's duties and responsibilities as well.

### 5A.4.1 GENERAL CARE CHECKLIST FOR THE ELDERLY

**1.**      **Housekeeping**

_____      Needs help with all housekeeping chores.
_____      Does not participate in any housekeeping chores.
_____      Performs certain housekeeping chores satisfactory
_____      Maintains house in good order but requires help occasionally

**2.**      **Food Preparation**

_____      Needs help in preparing meals at all times.
_____      Prepares adequate meals with some help.
_____      Heats and serves meals prepared by others.
_____      Can prepare meals with no help.

**3.**      **Transportation**

_____      Needs a companion to travel by bus.
_____      Arranges transportation (taxi, car) on his own.
_____      Cannot travel by bus.
_____      Drives own car.

**4.**      **Finances**

_____      Cannot manage own money.
_____      Manages day to day expenses but needs help with major purchases and monthly bank reconciliation.
_____      Manages financial matters independently.

**5.**      **Telephone/Correspondence**

_____      Can answer the phone but cannot dial out.
_____      Needs help in making calls or writing correspondence.
_____      Can use the phone and write letters without any help.

## 5A.4.2 PERSONAL CARE CHECKLIST FOR THE ELDERLY

1. **Medications**

    _____ Cannot take medications without help.

    _____ Needs to be reminded when to take medications.

    _____ Does not need any help (when, how) in taking medication.

2. **Physical Movement**

    _____ Needs help in moving around the house.

    _____ Needs some kind of aid (wheelchair, cane, companion) when moving in or out the house

    _____ Does not need any assistance in walking or moving about.

3. **Feeding**

    _____ Requires help in feeding self.

    _____ Requires some help in feeding self with certain kinds of food.

    _____ Can feed self without assistance.

4. **Grooming**

    _____ Needs total grooming at all times.

    _____ Needs help in grooming (remains well-groomed after).

    _____ Grooms self adequately but requires some help in using aids (shaver, hair dryer).

    _____ Does not require any help.

5. **Toileting**

    _____ Has no bowel control.

    _____ Has no bladder control.

    _____ Has bowel or bladder accidents once or twice a week.

    _____ Needs to be reminded to use toilet.

    _____ Has no bowel or bladder difficulty.

6. **Dressing**

    _____ Needs help in dressing or undressing.

    _____ Dresses or undresses self with minimum assistance.

    _____ Dresses or undresses self independently.

7. **Bathing**

    _____ Cannot wash self or does not wash self.

    _____ Can only wash face and hands.

    _____ Needs help in getting in or out of bath tub.

    _____ Needs help in getting in or out of shower.

    _____ Can bathe, wash and clean self without help.

It is important for the caregiver to note the date for example when the elderly requires constant help in a task or activity which was not checked previously as the family or family doctor may find the information useful in maintaining care.

## 5A.5 AGING, NUTRITION, AND MEAL PREPARATION

### 5-2

Maintaining an adequate nutritional intake is very important for the aging person, particularly to one who is socially, physically, and mentally ill. Improper food intake may be responsible for many complaints such as general fatigue, moodiness, and other emotional symptoms. In general, seniors drink less fluids and characteristically develop an intense liking for sugary foods. The deficiency mainly lies in inadequate intake of protein, calcium, and essential vitamins.

The aging person may not have the motivation for adequate meal planning and preparation. As a result, the person falls into a vicious cycle of poor nutrition intake which in turn leads to lowered energy level and can cause lack of appetite.

### 5A.5.1 FACTORS THAT AFFECT POOR NUTRITION INTAKE

| | |
|---|---|
| **Limited Income.** | Low budget may make it hard to buy amounts and the right kinds of food. Rent and utilities may eat up a major portion of the budget. Not proper packaging of meat and food may not motivate an aging person to prepare food properly. |
| **Inadequate Dentition.** | May cause chewing problems. Denture wearers may be unable to chew meats or fresh vegetables and fruits thus may restrict diets to soft and starchy foods. |
| **Fewer active taste-buds. (taste).** | Diminished acuity of sight, smell, and lessened motor skills may contribute to a deficient intake of food. |
| **Reduction.** | Reduced quantity of enzymes and gastric acidity may cause absorption difficulties. |
| **Loneliness.** | Unhappiness, fear, anxiety or living alone, may also affect the appetite and therefore food intake. |

| | |
|---|---|
| **Obesity.** | An inadequate protein intake may pose problem. Usually as people get older, their activity level decreases but not their food intake. |
| **Metabolic Rate.** | As the aging process takes place, basal metabolic rate decreases with a corresponding decrease in caloric needs. On the other hand, protein intake is of considerable importance due to the activity status of the person. The thing to remember, however, is the gradual loss of appetite or active food intake results in actual loss of protein and leads to further inactivity. |
| **Digestion.** | Because the process of digestion slows down with age, the elderly's meal size and its frequency must be adjusted. Proper amount of food intake depends on the energy and physical activities of the aging person. Hence, a dietary plan for the senior must be individualized based on the senior's activity and exercise needs. In addition, when planning a diet for the aged, the person's food custom must likewise be considered. It is simply useless to recommend changes for an improved diet without due regards to his/her socioeconomic, educational, religious, and cultural factors. |

## 5A.5.2 FOOD GROUPS AND NUTRITION INTAKE

Taken in Module 4.

## 5A.6        AGING, ILLNESSES AND DISEASES

### 5A.6.1 INDICATORS OF ILLNESSES

Following are indicators of illnesses for the elderly which demands immediate attention from the caregiver to avoid later complications:

| | |
|---|---|
| **Confusion.** | The start of confusion is not caused by just becoming old. Confusion maybe the result of side effects of medication, infection, depression, head injury, physical illness, or discomforts. |
| **Fever or elevated body temperature.** | This indicates that there is something wrong with the physical body or that an infection is present. Seniors have a hard time tolerating fever because it is usually accompanied by aches in joints and muscles, poor appetite, confusion, and to a certain extent, shortness of breath. |
| **Loss of Appetite.** | This is almost always present in any type of illness. It may indicate infection, depression, heart failure and aches (head, stomach, muscles and joints). |
| **Weight Gain or Weight Loss.** | May indicate some chronic problems such as diabetes, heart failure, poor nutrition, and lack of exercise. |
| **Shortness of Breath/Rapid Breathing.** | Breathing problems among seniors may indicate lung or bronchial disorders as well as diabetes and heart conditions. |
| **Stomach Pain/ Abdominal Pain.** | Serious conditions such as appendicitis and heart problems may result if this is not attended to. Common also is too much gas or problems with the bowel and bladder. |
| **Chest Pain.** | Heart attacks and abdominal problems may cause chest pain. Symptoms may include shortness of breath, aches, a feeling of indigestion and confusion. |
| **Incontinence or the loss of bladder control.** | This may include the loss or weakening of the nerve supply to the bladder, blockage of bladder outflow resulting in overflow, weakness of the bladder or urethra support, infection of the bladder and some medications. Physical mobility can also pose as a cause when the elderly cannot readily make the trip to the toilet as often as he needs to. Dementia and stroke may also affect the nervous system regulating the bladder control. Many types of incontinence can be improved. |

| | |
|---|---|
| | **Tips and hints:**<br>• Encourage the elderly to empty his bladder frequently and at scheduled times – for example: every two or three hours.<br>• Talk to the senior into having a urinal or a bedpan at the bedside to avoid accidents in bed.<br>• Arrange for a bedroom that is closer to the toilet.<br>• As a result of paralysis, the bladder may leak constantly, so it may be necessary to know how to use a catheter inserted through the urethra. The process is fairly easy to learn and safe to use. To prevent accidents from happening in bed, adult diapers can be purchased at some drugstores or specialty stores. |
| **Bowel Problems.** | "I can move the world if I can move my bowel" is the embodiment of how many seniors feel about bowel movement. There are many factors that affect bowel movement and cause constipation. Ranking high are inadequate food and fluid intake, not enough fiber in the diet, inactivity, infection, colon and rectal disorders, inadequate opportunities to use the toilet and certain medications.<br><br>**Tips and hints:**<br>• Exercise regularly by walking and moving various parts of the body in order to increase circulation and mobility.<br>• Eat proper food and take extra fiber in your diet.<br>• Use the toilet as necessary and don't hold urine or bowel movement for any length of time. If you need to go, GO!<br>• Consult your doctor for many of the over the counter medications that you take. Ask the doctor also, when he prescribes, whether the medication could affect your bowel movement so that you can take extra precaution.<br>• Avoid laxatives as much as possible because it leads to dependency and can have serious side effects.<br><br>The aging person may not have the motivation for adequate meal planning and preparation. As a result, the person falls into a vicious cycle of poor nutritional intake which in turn leads to lowered energy level and causes of lack of appetite. |

## 5A.6.2 FACTORS THAT AFFECT POOR NUTRITION INTAKE

See Topic 5A.5.1

## 5A.6.3 AGING AND DISABILITY

As we reach our retirement age, we may start experiencing restriction or lack of ability to perform an activity in the manner or within the range considered normal for a healthy young adult. This topic then is better discussed in a special module for special needs persons.

## 5A.6.4 COMMON ILLNESSES AND DISEASES OF THE ELDERLY (GLOSSARY)

### 1.    Alzheimer's Disease
- Alzheimer's Disease is a culmination of several disorders.
- Most commonly recognized as the gradual loss of brain cells. The rate at which this degradation can take years (3-20).
- Memory and thinking skills are targeted first and eventually other parts of the brain start to deteriorate.

### 2.    Anemia
- The blood in your body contains three main types of cells; one in particular called red blood cells, transports oxygen (using Hemoglobin) to various parts of your body. Oxygen is an important component of energy generation in cells.
- Anemia occurs when there is an insufficient amount of red blood cells in the body.
- The most recognizable symptom of anemia is constantly feeling tired.
- Other symptoms include:
  a. Fatigue
  b. Shortness of breath
  c. Dizziness or fainting
  d. Pale skin
  e. Rapid heart beat
  f. Feeling cold
  g. Sadness and depression

### 3.    Arthritis (Osteoathritis, Rheumatoid, Gout)
- The most basic definition of Arthritis is joint inflammation which is marked by burning, pain, swelling and redness.
- Osteoathritis, rheumatoid, and gout are the three most common forms of arthritis.

  #### a. Osteoarthritis
  ➢ The break down of the cartilage inside the joints.

> ➢ This is most commonly found on fingers, elbow, knees, shoulder, and the wrists. Osteoarthritis is usually the result of overstress on these joints.
> ➢ Symptoms include steady pain in the joint, stiffness following periods of inactivity, swelling or tenderness of one or more joints, crunching feeling (feeling of two bones rubbing of two bones).

### b. Rheumatoid
> ➢ It is the lining around the joints called synovium.
> ➢ Symptoms include joints being affected feel warm, swollen, or tender, fatigue, lumps of tissue under the skin called rheumatoid nodules and pain other than in the joints.

### c. Gout
> ➢ It is a form of arthritis which is the result of a build up of uric acid in the body. Excessive uric acid causes build up around the joints.
> ➢ In time, the uric acid develops into needle-like crystals in the joints that form acute gout.
> ➢ Most common causes of gout are excessive alcohol intake, offal foods (liver, tripe, kidney, and tongue), shellfish, and excessive weight loss.

## 4.     Atherosclerosis
- Atherosclerosis is a process in which plaque builds up on the inner lining of arteries. Plaque consists of deposits of fatty substances, cholesterol, cellular waste products, calcium, and other products. As a person gets older, the plaque hardens and causes a myriad of health problems.
- Blockage due to plaque can cause high blood pressure and blood clots. If a blockage occurs at a blood vessel that feeds the heart, it will cause a heart attack. A stroke occurs when a blood vessel that feeds the brain is blocked.
- Most common cause of atherosclerosis area elevated levels of cholesterol and triglyceride (tri-GLIS'er-id) in the blood, high blood pressure, tobacco smoke and diabetes.

## 5.     Cancer
- In general, cancer is defined as uncontrolled growth and spread abnormal cells in the body. Genes are found in cells, which control cell growth, function, and cell reproduction. When the genes get damaged, their instructions are altered and may cause the cell to reproduce uncontrollably.
- Causes of some gene damage include smoking, poor diet, lack of exercise, and unprotected exposure to the sun.

### 6. *Chronic Obstructive Pulmonary Disease (COPD)*

- Chronic Obstructive Pulmonary Disease is a generic term for lung disease. Most common cases are Chronic Bronchitis and Emphysema.

#### a. Chronic bronchitis
  - ➢ It occurs when there is an excessive production of mucus causing airway obstruction and bronchial lining scaring in the lungs. Symptoms include chronic cough, increased mucus, frequent clearing of the throat and shortness of breathe.

#### b. Emphysema
  - ➢ Occurs when the air sacks in the lung loose their ability stretch and recoil. This causes the air sacks to weaken and break. The lung tissue looses its elasticity and the exchange of carbon dioxide and oxygen in the lungs is impaired.
  - ➢ The effects of emphysema are irreversible.
  - ➢ Symptoms of emphysema include cough, shortness of breath and a limited exercise tolerance.

### 7. Congestive Heart Failure

- This is caused by the insufficient blood circulation by the heart to supply oxygen to the body. This results in the blood to flow backwards from the heart and congesting the lungs. The heart compensates by over working itself, which could lead to more cardiac problems. Results of this compensation include an enlarged heart, thickening of the heart muscle wall, abnormally fast heartbeat, and kidney malfunctions.
- Causes of congestive heart failure include coronary heart disease, high blood pressure, heart attacks, and lung disease.

### 8. Constipation

- Tiny amounts of dry and hard bowel movement. Constipation may cause difficult and even painful bowel movements.
- Symptoms include bloating, feeling uncomfortable, and feeling sluggish.
- Causes of constipation include not enough fiber in the diet, not enough liquids, lack of exercise, medications, irritable bowel syndrome, changes in life or routine such as pregnancy, older age, and travel, abuse of laxatives, ignoring the urge to have a bowel movement, stroke (by far the most common), problems with the colon and rectum and problems with intestinal function (chronic idiopathic constipation).

### 9. Decubitus Ulcer

- Decubitus ulcer is a pressure sore or more commonly known as a bed sore. Sores may appear mild pink or as deep wounds that can extend into bone or even through organs and are similar to burn wounds.
- Usual causes of decubitus ulcers is the friction due to rubbing on objects such as bed sheets, casts, braces, and prolonged exposure to the cold.
- Most prone areas of the body are areas where skin just lies over bone such as elbows, knees, and heels are just a few. In these areas, blood circulation is easily blocked and tissue starts to die.
- Simplest prevention method is changing positions every couple of hours.

### 10. Dehydration

- The lack of water and essential body salt ions (Potassium and Sodium ions) in the body. Minimum number of water and ions results in the impairment of vital organs such as the kidneys, brain and the heart.
- Below are symptoms of mild, moderate ,and severe cases of dehydration

| *Mild* | **Moderate** | *Severe* |
|---|---|---|
| ▪ Thirst | ▪ Very dry mouth membranes | ▪ All signs of moderate dehydration |
| ▪ Dry lips | ▪ Sunken eyes | ▪ Rapid, weak pulse (more than 100 at rest). |
| ▪ Slightly dry mouth membranes | ▪ Sunken fontanelle (soft spot) on infant's head | ▪ Cold hands and feet |
| | ▪ Skin doesn't bounce back quickly when lightly pinched and released | ▪ Rapid breathing |
| | | ▪ Blue lips |
| | | ▪ Confusion, lethargy, difficult to arouse |

### 11. Depression

- Depressive disorder is an illness that involves ones body, mood and thoughts. It can affect the way one eats, sleeps, and how one thinks about themselves. There are 3 major types of depression.

#### a. Dysthymia

➢ It is a less severe form of depression. Chronic symptoms are not disabling but may be long term and interfere with work, sleep, eating, and enjoying things that were one pleasurable.

#### b. Major Depression

➢ Similar to dysythymia but has a disabling attacks which may occur more than once in ones lifetime.

> Symptoms include the following:
>> a. Persistently sad anxious, or "empty" mood
>> b. Feelings of hopelessness
>> c. Pessimism
>> d. Feelings of guilt, worthlessness, helplessness
>> e. Loss of interest or pleasure in hobbies and activities that were once enjoyed, including sex
>> f. Decreased energy
>> g. Fatigue/ being "slowed down"
>> h. Difficulty concentrating, remembering, making decisions
>> i. Insomnia, early-morning awakening, or oversleeping
>> j. Appetite and/or weight loss or overeating and weight gain
>> k. Thoughts of death or suicide, suicide attempts
>> l. Restlessness
>> m. Irritability
>> n. Persistent physical symptoms that do not respond to treatment, such as headaches, digestive disorders, and chronic pains

### c. Bipolar Disorder
> Also called manic depressive illness, characterized by periods of high (manias) and low (depression) moods. Mood changes can be sporadic but mostly gradual.
> Symptoms of manias include:
>> a. Abnormal or excessive elation
>> b. Unusual irritability
>> c. Decreased need for sleep
>> d. Grandiose notions
>> e. Increased talking
>> f. Racing thoughts
>> g. Increased sexual desire
>> h. Markedly increased energy
>> i. Poor judgment
>> j. Inappropriate social behavior

## 12. Diabetes Mellitus
- This results from the inability of the pancreas to produce insulin (hormone needed for the metabolism of sugar and starches) or the ineffectiveness of the insulin resulting to high blood sugar content.
- Complications due to diabetes mellitus include damage of blood vessels in the retina, loss of metabolic control, kidney failure, heart disease, and easy ulceration of the limbs.
- There are two types of diabetes:

### a. Type 1 Diabetes
> Lack of insulin production by the pancreas which results in the person having to take insulin (always taken by injection, not by mouth). Symptoms include:
>> a. Excessive urination
>> b. Constant thirst
>> c. Weight loss
>> d. Tiredness

### b. Type 2 Diabetes
> Inability of the body to react to insulin when released. 90% of insulin cases are type 2 diabetes. Symptoms of type 2 diabetes are the same as type 1 and are more subtle, and the early symptoms are not visible.
> Diagnosis of Type 2 diabetes is evident only after several years of the condition.

## 13.   Diarrhea

- Loose bowel movement that has a watery consistency that occurs more than three times a day. Time span may be a day or two and prolonged diarrhea could be a sign of something more serious.
- Common symptoms of diarrhea are abdominal pain, bloating, urgent use of the washroom, bloody stools, and dehydration.
- Some common causes of diarrhea are:
  a. Bacterial infections by consuming contaminated food or water. Bacteria such as *Campylobacter, Salmonella, Shigella,* and *Escherichia col* causes diarrhea.
  b. Many viruses cause diarrhea, including rotavirus, Norwalk virus, cytomegalovirus, herpes simplex virus, and viral hepatitis.
  c. Food intolerances due to an inability to digest a food compound, eg. lactose in milk
  d. Parasites such as *Giardia lamblia, Entamoeba histolytica,* and *Cryptosporidium,* when injested through food or water and settle in the digestive system causes diarrhea.
  e. Reaction to medicines, such as antibiotics, blood pressure medications, and antacids containing magnesium.
  f. Intestinal diseases, like inflammatory bowel disease or celiac disease.
  g. Functional bowel disorders, such as irritable bowel syndrome, in which the intestines do not work normally.

## 14.   Dementia
- The loss of brain functions as the result of disease or injury. Such functions include decision-making, judgment, spatial orientation, thinking, reasoning and verbal communication.

- Behavioral changes occur such as trouble with dressing, changed eating behavior, personality changes, and the inability to do routine activities. Some effects of dementia is reversible however dementia due to the onset of Alzheimer's disease or multiple strokes.

## 15.   Epilepsy
- Epilepsy is the condition in which multiple seizures occur. A seizure is the temporary interruption of most or all of the brains functions such as consciousness, awareness, control of movement, and body posture.
- Having one seizure in one's lifetime does not suggest epilepsy.
- Some diseases such as Cerebral Palsy, Meningitis, and Encephalitis cause epilepsy. Brain trauma, strokes, and tumors are also known to cause epilepsy.

## 16.   Goiter
- A non-cancerous swelling of the thyroid gland. Simplest form of goiter is formed as a result of a lack of thyroid hormone to the body, the thyroid compensates by increasing production of the hormone by enlarging itself.

### *Endemic goiter*
The most common form of simple goiter is the lack of iodine in the diet.
Symptoms include:
    a.  Neck lumps
    b.  Breathing difficulties (wheezing from the lungs)
    c.  Difficulties swallowing (swelling of the esophagus)
    d.  Dizziness when arms are raised above the shoulder

## 17.   Hemorrhoids
- Inflammation and swelling of the veins around the lower rectum.
- Causes of hemorrhoids include the inability to have bowel movements, pregnancy, diarrhea, and anal intercourse.
- External cases of hemorrhoids have symptoms of painful swells and lumps around the anus.
- Internal hemorrhoids have the basic symptom of having bright red covered fecal matter or bright red deposits on toilet paper.

## 18.   Hepatitis
- There are wide range of Hepatitis viruses. All have the common property that they are viruses that attack the liver.

### a. Hepatitis A
> ➢ Hepatitis A virus causes Hepatitis A.
> ➢ Hepatitis A virus is spread by the ingestion of items that have been contaminated by the fecal matter of a person with the virus.
> ➢ Symptoms include diarrhea, fever, nausea, fatigue, jaundice, abdominal pain, and loss of appetite.

### b. Hepatitis B
> ➢ Hepatitis B virus causes Hepatitis B.
> ➢ Hepatitis B is a much more serious disease and can lead to liver failure, liver cancer, and eventually death.
> ➢ The disease is spread by the exchange of bodily fluids from an infected person like sharing needles or unprotected sex.
> ➢ Hepatitis B has the same symptoms as Hepatitis A with the inclusion of joint pain.

There are two other forms of Hepatitis: Hepatitis C and Hepatitis D. Hepatitis D exists only in the presence of Hepatitis C.

## 19. Hypertension
- Also known as high blood pressure.
- High blood pressure is caused by various reasons ranging from narrowing of the arteries; increased heart beat, high volume of blood, and may be caused by other diseases.
- High blood pressure can lead to strokes, retinal damage, heart disease, and heart attacks.
- Symptoms of high blood pressure are blood pressure readings consistently higher than 140/90 mmHg.
- Preventive measures can be taken by increased physical activity, maintaining a reasonable weight, eating more fruits and vegetables, preparing foods with less salt, and drinking alcohol in moderation.

## 20. Lupus erythematosis
- Chronic Inflammation of the skin, joints, and internal organs.
- *Lupus erythematosis* is an autoimmune disease which is a malfunction of the body's own immune system where the immune system attacks the body it is trying to protect.
- Cause of the wrongful attack on the bodies organs is still unknown.
- Symptoms include:
  - a. Fever
  - b. Constant feeling of illness
  - c. Fatigue
  - d. Weight loss

e. Skin rash due to sensitivity to sunlight
f. Arthritis
g. Swollen glands
h. Nausea and vomiting
i. Bloody urine
j. Abdominal pain
k. Hair loss
l. Mouth sores

## 21. Meningitis

- Inflammation of the brain lining called the meninges. Inflammation can be due to viral or bacterial infection.

### a. Bacterial Meningitis
  ➤ Bacterial Meningitis is caused by meningococcal and pneumococcal bacteria.
  ➤ Common means of bacterial spread include kissing, coughing, and sneezing.
  ➤ If left untreated, it may lead to handicaps or even brain damage.

### b. Viral Meningitis
  ➤ Less serious than bacterial meningitis.
  ➤ It is caused by enteroviruses and is spread through coughing or sneezing. However, viral meningitis is also caused by other diseases such as herpes, polio, and chickenpox.
  ➤ Symptoms of viral meningitis is similar to bacterial meningitis with the inclusion of diarrhea, and salivary gland swelling.

## 22. Myocardial Infarction

- Also known as "heart attacks."
- Involves the death of heart cells due to lack of oxygen and other nutrients.
- This is the result of plaque blockage of the arterial wall.
- Injured heart muscle cells after a heart attack can heal however scar tissue is formed which can prevent the heart from function regularly.

## 23. Pneumonia

- General term for infection of the lungs. Infection can be bacterial, viral, fungal, or parasitic.
- Pneumonia bacteria can actually be found in the throat of a healthy person. When the immune system is weaken, these bacteria spread and cause problems in the lungs. Weakening of the immune system can be due to malnutrition, old age, or other illnesses.
- Most common bacterial Pneumonia is streptococcus pneumonia. Symptoms include high fever, rapid breathing and increased heart rate. Lips and nails

may appear blue due to lack of oxygen.

- Viral Pneumonia can be caused by viruses such as influenza, which invades the lungs resulting in fluid in the lungs. Symptoms include dry cough, fever, headache, muscle pain, shortness of breath, and blueness of the lips.

## 24.    Pulmonary Embolism

- Arterial blockage in the lungs due to air, fat, tumor tissue, or blood clots which can lead to sudden death.
- Most affected are inactive persons, oral contraceptive users, people with heart attacks or strokes, and people who have received heart surgery.
- Symptoms include:
    a.  Coughing with bloody spit
    b.  Sudden shortness of breath
    c.  Fainting
    d.  Dizziness
    e.  Splinting of the ribs while breathing
    f.  Chest pain
    b.  Rapid heart beat
    c.  Sweating

## 25.    Pulmonary Tuberculosis

- Infection of the Mycobacterium tuberculosis bacteria which initially attacks the lungs and can spread to other parts of the body.
- Mycobacterium is spread through the air by coughing and sneezing by an infected person.
- Symptoms include:
    a.  Fatigue
    b.  Weight loss
    c.  Coughing out blood
    d.  High fever with sweating
    e.  Wheezing of the lungs
    f.  Excessive sweating
    g.  Chest pains
    h.  Difficulty with breathing

## 26.    Rheumatic Fever

- Prolonged untreated effects of an upper respiratory infection caused by type A streptococci.
- Rheumatic fever causes inflammation of the bodies connective tissue especially the joints, heart, brain, and the skin.
- Rheumatic fever can lead to Rheumatic heart disease, which is the damage of the heart valves.
- Symptoms of Rheumatic fever include:

a. Fever
b. Mild arthritis
c. Abdominal pain
d. Skin rashes that appear like coils
e. Uncoordinated movements in the face feet and hands
f. Shortness of breath

## 27. Severe Acute Respiratory Syndrome (SARS)

- Serious Respiratory disease first reported in East and South East Asia.
- Infected persons will initially have flu like symptoms that lead to pneumonia and difficulty of breathing. Death can result, however it is relative to age and if contracted in the presence of other ailments.
- Little is known about the transmission of the disease but being in the vicinity of a person of SARS increases risk of infection.
- Symptoms of the initial flu-like conditions which last for 2-10 days which include high fever, shortness of breath or difficulties in breathing.
- Other symptoms include:
  a. Headaches
  b. Muscular stiffness
  c. Diarrhea

## 28. Transient Ischemic Attack

- Transient stroke attack that only lasts for a few minutes due to an interruption of blood flow to the brain.
- Symptoms are temporary and disappear within an hour of the attack to 24 hours after the attack.
- Symptoms include:
  a. Numbness on the face, arms, and leg
  b. Difficulty in talking and comprehension of speech
  c. Loss of balance and coordination

## 29. Urinary Tract Infection

- Microorganisms like *Chlamydia* and *Mycoplasma* and bacteria from the digestive tract cling to the urethra wall and begin to multiply.
- Most common bacterial infection is due to E. Coli bacteria, which is present in the colon. From the urethra wall, the bacteria can move up to the bladder, and eventually to the kidneys if left untreated.
- Symptoms of Urinary Tract infection include:
  a. Painful urination
  b. A burning sensation in the bladder and urethra during urination,
  c. Constant feeling of the urge to urinate but little urine is passed
  d. milky or bloody urine
- An infection in women causes a feeling of pressure on the pubic bone.
- Men have symptoms of fullness in the rectum.

# 5A.7 QUESTIONS

1. Define/describe the process of aging.

2. What are the phases of aging? Describe it briefly.

3. Name the four types of aging and its characteristics?

4. List at least 10 various roles a caregiver has to perform for the elderly?

5. What are the rights of the elderly?

6. What are the needs and activities of the elderly?

7. Give five common diseases of the elderly? Describe each briefly.

8. How should a caregiver handle an elderly with a poor self-image or low self-esteem?

9. State five anecdotes that show the characteristics of an aging person.

10. Enumerate five factors that affect an elderly's nutrition intake.

11. Enumerate five common indicators of illnesses among the elderly that demands immediate attention from the caregiver?

12. What preventive measures can be observed against the occurrence of hypertension among the elderly?

13. Describe dementia and the behavioral changes among the elderly.

14. What is diabetes mellitus?

15. What is bipolar disorder? Give five symptoms.

# MODULE
# 5B
## Disability

*Julie V. Kallal*

# CONTENTS OF MODULE 5B

| **5B.1** | **INTRODUCTION** |
|---|---|

## GENERAL TYPES OF DISABILITIES

**Disability**   The lack of an ability we would like to have, presumably in order to do something we wish to do, and therefore to experience a critical mismatch in a certain range of tasks.

Also results from an impairment and is defined as any restriction or lack of ability to perform an activity in the manner within the range considered normal for a human being.

Disability has 2 types, as follows:

**Partial**   The loss or reduction of working capacity, productivity, or ability to learn. Loss or reduction of biological learning capacity due to the virtually permanent consequences of a pathological event casually related to an occupational accident or disease.

**Total**   If the disability is total and absolute, the assessment will naturally be 100% - however, the terms "total" and "absolute" should not be taken literally, for it is obvious that totally disabled persons also include those who are merely unable to engage in any gainful activity, thus cannot take advantage of the small portion of capacity that remains to them (e.g. a blind person should always be considered totally disabled even if he manages to find some useful occupation).

## 5B.2             TERMS OF DISABILITY

| IMPAIRMENT | DISABILITY | HANDICAP |
|---|---|---|
| ➢ Any temporary or permanent loss or abnormality of psychological, physiological or anatomical structure or function.<br><br>*Ex: language, hearing, vision, skeletal, psychological* | ➢ Results from an impairment and is defined as any restriction or lack of ability to perform an activity in the manner or within the range considered normal for a human being.<br><br>*Ex: speaking, seeing, dressing, feeding, behavioral* | ➢ The disadvantage for a given individual, resulting from an impairment or disability that limits or prevents the fulfillment's of a role that is considered normal for that individual depending upon age, sex, social and cultural factors.<br><br>*Ex: orientation, physical independence, social independence* |

**Kinds of Impairments:**

**A. Mental Impairment**
(Intellectual and psychological impairments)

1. Mental retardation
2. Psychosis
3. Alcoholism
4. Chronic depression or anxiety
5. Convulsive Disorders

**B. Physical Impairment**

1. Language
2. Aural
3. Ocular
4. Vascular
5. Skeletal
6. Disfiguring impairments

# 5B.3                                        CAUSES OF DISABILITIES

## VARIOUS KINDS OF DISABILITIES

Behavior disabilities                Locomotor disabilities            Particular skill disabilities
Communication disabilities           Body disposition disabilities
Personal Care disabilities           Situational disabilities

### COMMON CAUSES OF DISABILITY AND DEATH

#### *Age Group of 65 and Over*

The following are the major causes of disability and death from long term illness which are common in the older age group:
- Heart disease – except rheumatic
- Hypertensive vascular disease
- Cancer
- Accidents
- Pneumonia
- Diabetes
- Rheumatic fever and rheumatic heart
- Liver and gallbladder

#### *Among People Who Usually Work*

The three leading causes of chronic limitation affecting ability to work:
- Heart condition                                14%
- Arthritis and rheumatism                       12%
- Impairment of the back or spine                11%

#### *Among Children*

- Malnutrition
- Poor environmental sanitation
- Communicable diseases
- Infection
- Accident
- Absence of information about proper health measures
- Lack of proper stimulation and early education among children
- Stresses and emotional disturbances

These causes in children may result in:
- Blindness
- Mental illness
- Mentally subnormal
- Hearing impaired
- Physically handicapped

*Examples of Impairment, Disability, and Handicap:*

### 1. A boy is involved in vehicular collision and one leg has to be amputated above the knee.

| Impairment | Disability | Handicap |
|---|---|---|
| Loss of leg | Decreased ability to walk and affected the manner of walking | <ul><li>Decreased ability to work</li><li>To enjoy normal social activities, sports, dancing</li><li>To have social relationships</li></ul> |

### 2. Severely malnourished child.

| Impairment | Disability | Handicap |
|---|---|---|
| Malnutrition | Inability to crawl, walk, run, stand and learn | Decreased ability to enjoy social activities and social relationships |

### 3. Married man with excessive daily intake of liquor.

| Impairment | Disability | Handicap |
|---|---|---|
| Disturbance of brain function, impaired sensation in hands and feet, liver damage, etc., due to too much drinking | Lack of judgment and motivation | Inability to work, decreased output, inability to maintain economic necessities of life, and disturbed social relations. |

### 4. Mentally retarded boy with no education.

| Impairment | Disability | Handicap |
|---|---|---|
| Brain damage | <ul><li>Abnormally low intelligence</li><li>Slowness in acquisition</li><li>Inability to read, write or make simple calculations</li></ul> | Unable to work and disturbed social relationships |

### 5. A person with Leprosy for several years.

| Impairment | Disability | Handicap |
|---|---|---|
| Injury to the nerves | <ul><li>Inability to feel or loss of sensation</li><li>Decreased mobility and motor skills</li><li>Paralysis</li></ul> | <ul><li>Inability to have normal social relationships</li><li>Inability to find work</li></ul> |

## 5B.4            PHYSICAL IMPAIRMENTS

### 5B.4.1 OCULAR DISABILITY

| | |
|---|---|
| **Symptoms** | Inability to see includes visual acuity of one or both eyes caused by cataracts, Injury, glaucoma, diabetes, and other unknown causes.<br><br>Difficulty with seeing can be mild, moderate and severe. A person is considered blind if he sees very little or nothing. Some, however, can see the difference between light and dark or day and night, but cannot see shapes of things. Others can see shapes of large objects but none of the details. Some children are born blind. Others become blind during early childhood or later in life as a result of accidents or diseases.<br><br>Not all blind people have eyes that look different. Their eyes may look clear and normal. The damage may be behind the eyes or in part of the brain. |
| **Signs** | 1. Eyes or eyelids are red, have pus and continually form tears.<br>2. Eyes look dull, cloudy, have sores or other obvious problems.<br>3. One or both pupils look gray or white.<br>4. Has difficulty seeing after the sun sets (night blindness).<br>5. Among children:<br>   • By 3 months the child's eyes still do not follow an object or light that is moved in front of him<br>   • By 3 months the infant does not reach for things held in front of him, unless the things make sound or touch him<br>   • Child squints or tips head to look at things.<br>   • Child slower to use hands, move about, or walk than other children and seems clumsy and bumps into things.<br>   • Child takes little in brightly colored objects, pictures, books or he put such materials very close to his face.<br>   • Eyes "cross" or one eye turns in or out, moves differently from the other. Note: some eye crossing is normal up to 6 months.<br>   • In school, the child can't see the blackboard, nor read small prints, and gets tired or headaches when he reads. |

## 5B.4.2AURAL DISABILITY

| | |
|---|---|
| **Symptoms** | Hearing problems may be classified as mild or severe and are caused by congenital (existing at birth) absence of hearing, perforated eardrum, accidents and other unknown causes. Some are completely deaf, meaning, they cannot hear at all, and some are partly deaf. |
| **Signs** | Parents or caregivers may notice early that a child cannot hear, because he does not turn his head or respond, even to loud sounds. A child may show surprise or turn his head to a loud noise but not to softer noises. He may respond to a low-pitched sound like thunder or a drum but not to a high pitched sound like a whistle. |

## 5B.4.3MUSCULOSKELETAL DISABILITY

Specific types include lower limbs disability caused by poliomyelitis, paraplegia due to illness or accidents and other unknown causes.

| | | |
|---|---|---|
| **1.** | **Polio** | Paralysis begins when the child is small, often during illness like a bad cold with fever and sometimes diarrhea. Paralysis may affect any muscles of the body, but is most common in the legs. Some muscles may be only partly weakened, others may get by limping. In time, the limb may not be able to straighten all the way due to shortening or contractures of certain muscles. The muscles and bones of the affected limb become thinner than other limb. The affected limb does not grow as fast and so is shorter. Unaffected arms or legs often become extra strong to make up for parts that are weak. Intelligence and mind are not affected. |
| **2.** | **Muscular Dystrophy** | A progressive disease, the condition weakens month by month and year by year. The person becomes weaker and weaker.<br><br>**Signs:**<br>• Mostly affects males (rarely females).<br>• Often brothers or male relatives have similar problems.<br>• First signs appear around the ages of 3 to 5 years. The child may seem awkward or clumsy or may begin to walk using his tiptoes (because he cannot put his feet flat on the floor. He runs strangely and falls often).<br>• The condition becomes progressively worse. Muscle weakness first affects feet, fronts of the thigh, hips, belly, shoulders, and elbows. Later it affects hands, face, and neck muscles.<br>• By age 19, the child may no longer be able to walk.<br>• He may then develop a severe curve of the spine.<br>• Heart and breathing muscles also get weak. The child usually dies before his 20th birthday usually from heart failure or pneumonia. |
| **3.** | **Contractures** | Contractures are limbs that can no longer be straightened. When an arm or a leg is in a bent position for a long period of time, some of the muscles become shorter, so that the limb cannot fully straighten. Shortened muscles may then hold a joint in a straight position only therefore the joint can no longer be bent. Contractures can develop in any joint of the body and are progressive. |

| 4. Cerebral Palsy | Means "brain paralysis". It is disability that affects movement and body position. The brain may be damaged long before the baby is born, while the baby is being born, or while the baby is still very young. The whole brain may not all be affected but usually the parts that control movements are affected. |

### How to recognize Cerebral Palsy (early signs)

- At birth, a baby with cerebral palsy is often limp and floppy, or may even seem normal.
- Baby may or may jot breathe right away at birth, and may turn blue and floppy. Delayed breathing is a common cause of brain damage.
- Slow development. Compared to other children, the child is slow to hold up his head, to sit, or to move around.
- Baby may not use his hands or uses only one hand and does not begin to use both hands.
- Feeding problems. The child may have difficulty sucking, swallowing, or chewing. He may choke or gag often. Even as the child gets bigger, these and other feeding problems may continue.
- Difficulties in taking care of the baby or young child. His body may stiffen when he is carried, dressed, or washed or during play. Later, he may not learn to feed or dress himself, to wash, to use toilet by himself, and to play with others. Baby seems to always have a sudden stiffening of the body, being floppy, or simply 'falling all over place'.

- Watch for the body being so limp that his head may seem to fall off or sudden stiffening like a board. Hugging and carrying may seem impossible.
- Extreme behavior. The child may cry a lot, may become very irritable, may be really fussy; or he may be very quiet and passive and becomes weaker and weaker.

## Jason's Case

Jason spent the first years of his life crawling because one leg was paralyzed. Because he could not stand, he kept his hip and knee bent and his foot in a tiptoe position.

In time, he could not straighten his hip, knee nor bend his foot up. He has developed a hip contracture, a knee contracture a "tiptoe" contracture of the ankle. Because of the contractures, Jason could not stand or walk, even with a brace.

Remember, contractures develop whenever a limb or joint is not moved regularly through its full range of motion. Therefore, it is important to exercise different body parts of people who are bedridden.

## 5B.5      COMMON BIRTH DEFECTS

### 5B.5.1 CAUSES OF BIRTH DEFECTS

There are many causes for birth defects.  In many cases, the cause of birth defects is not known.  However, a defect may be caused by one of the following.

| | |
|---|---|
| **Poor Nutrition** | During pregnancy. |
| **Genetic (hereditary)** | Sometimes certain defects run in the family. For this reason, birth defects are more common in children whose parents are closely related and who therefore carry the same defect factors. |
| **Medicines, pesticides, Chemicals, and poisons** | During the first three months in the womb, ababy is susceptible to all kinds of hazardous products that the mother may take , eat or drink. |
| **German Measles** | If the mother gets German Measles during the first three months of pregnancy, it can cause defects in the baby.  The usual defects may affect the senses (hearing and seeing), the brain (cerebral palsy and retardation) or the organs inside the body (heart / liver).  Sometimes the baby is born with "rubber band" like grooves on the limbs and deformed or missing fingers or limbs. |
| **Children born to mother 40 years of age or older** | Children  born to mothers 40 years of age or older are more likely to have **Down's Syndrome** and defects of the hands, feet or organs. Down's Syndrome is a congenital disorder characterized by moderate to severe mental retardation, a short, flattened skull and slanting eyes. |

### 5B.5.2 RESULTS OF BIRTH DEFECTS

#### *Amputation*

The term used for the loss of some part of the body.  Rarely are children born without one or both hands and feet.  More often, a person loses an arm, leg, hand or foot because of accidents, advanced bone infection or damaged tissues.

Deciding what to do for an amputee depends on a number of things, including age, the amount of amputation, cost of remediation and above all, what the amputee wants or accepts.

### Missing Both Hands

- The amputee may want and accept such devices as hooks or whatever can help him hold things better. A child with upper arm amputations from birth often learns to use his feet almost as well as his hands.

### Missing One Hand

- If the amputee was born without a hand and is given an artificial limb early, he will usually accept the limb and keep using it. In some cases, however, where some person was amputated as an older child or he has managed for a long time without an artificial limb, he may prefer to keep using the stump. The use of the artificial limb must be encouraged so that he can get used to it and rely less and less on his stump.

### Amputation Below the Knee (Missing one or both legs)

- The amputee is usually fitted with an artificial leg as soon as possible or in the case of a child, by one year of age. A growing child will need several replacements as he grows older, so extra care is usually requires during his adjustment periods.

### One Leg is Missing Above the Knee

- Depending on who is paying for the artificial limb, if the amputation happens early in life or the child is born with a missing leg, an artificial leg with no joint can be fitted up to age 10. Otherwise, a leg with a joint is preferable.

### Both Legs are Missing

- Early in life, the child will move about on short "stump" limbs. Later on, he may wish to try some artificial limbs and crutches. Usually though, a wheelchair is recommended.

### Spinal Cord and Other Back Deformities

- The backbone or spine is a chain of bones called vertebrae that connects that head to the hipbone. Separating each of the vertebra is a small cushion called disks. The backbone holds the body and head upright. It also encloses, in its hollow center, the spinal cord or trunk line of nerves connecting the brain to all parts of the body.

**Spinal Curve Injury**

- Usually results from an accident that breaks or severely damages the central nerve cord in the neck or back.

**Sideways Curve (Scoliosis)**

- An S-shaped curve may result from unequal paralysis of back muscles or from a hip tilt due to one shorter leg. Sometimes though, the cause is unknown.

**Rounded Back (Kyphosis)**

- A rounded back may result from weak back muscles or from poor posture (bent over position when standing or sitting.)

**Swayback (Lordosis)**

- A sway back may result from weak stomach muscles, from hip contractures, or from the way the child walks to make up for a weak leg or hip. Sharp bend or Bump in the Spine (Tuberculosis of the Backbone). Tuberculosis of the backbone may result from destruction of one or more vertebrae by tuberculosis infection.

### 5B.6.1 Mental Retardation

**Mental retardation** is a delay or slowness in a child's mental development. The child learns things more slowly than other children his age. He may be late at the beginning to move, smile, show interest in things, use his hands, sit, walk, speak, and understand. Mental retardation ranges from mild to severe.

*Mildly Retarded* persons take longer to learn certain skills but with help, they can grow up to care for themselves and to take active responsible parts in the community.

*Severely Retarded* persons, as they grow older, stay at the mental age of a baby or a young child. They will always need to be cared for in some ways.

Mental retardation cannot be cured, however, all mentally retarded can be helped to progress more quickly. The earlier special help or stimulation begins, the more ability and skills the retarded gain.

## 5B.6.2OTHER MENTAL IMPAIRMENTS

**Alcoholism**  Characterized by continued or habitual excessive and usually uncontrollable use of alcohol beverages.

**Anxiety**  A painful uneasiness of mind especially fear that something unpleasant or unfortunate experience will happen.

**Epilepsy**  A disorder of the nervous system characterized by chronic fits (repeated fits over a long period of time).

**Fits**  Also called seizures or convulsive disorders which are sudden, usually brief, periods of unconsciousness or changes in mental state, often with strange jerking movements.

**Meningitis**  Fits in a very ill child may be sign of Meningitis, for which immediate medical treatment is necessary.

**Mongolism**  A malformation present at birth in which the child has slanting eyes, a large tongue, and a broad, short flattened nose and is frequently of extremely low mentality.

**Psychosis**  Any of a class of serious mental disorders in which the mind cannot function normally and the ability to deal with reality is impaired or lost.

**Tetanus**  The spasms of Tetanus can be mistaken for fits. The jaw shuts tightly (lockjaw) and the body suddenly bends back.

## 5B.7 QUESTIONS

1. What is a disability?

2. What are the general types of disabilities? Give its brief description.

3. Differentiate impairment, disability, and handicap from each other.

4. Cite two examples each for impairment, disability, and handicap.

5. Enumerate three examples of physical impairment.

6. Give three examples of mental impairment

7. Name at least three common causes of disabilities for the following age groups: 65 and over; people who usually work; and children.

8. Provide the corresponding impairment, disability, and handicap for the situation below:

"A boy is involved in vehicular collision and one leg has to be amputated above the knee."

| Impairment | Disability | Handicap |
|------------|-----------|----------|
|            |           |          |

9. Provide the corresponding impairment, disability, and handicap for the situation below.

"Severely malnourished child."

| Impairment | Disability | Handicap |
|------------|-----------|----------|
|            |           |          |

10. Identify the corresponding impairment, disability, and handicap for the situation below.

"Married man with excessive daily intake of liquor."

| Impairment | Disability | Handicap |
|------------|-----------|----------|
|            |           |          |

11. What is an ocular disability?

12. Identify three signs of ocular disability.

13. Give three signs of ocular disability among children.

14. Identify three symptoms of ocular disability.

15. What are three signs of aural disability in a child?

16. Give four examples of musculoskeletal disability.

17. How is polio developed in an individual?

18. What is muscular dystrophy?

19. How progressive is the development of muscular dystrophy in an individual?

20. What are contractures?

21. Describe how contractures are formed?

22. How can contractures be prevented on bedridden patients?

23. What is cerebral palsy and how does it affect a baby?

24. What are the recognizable early signs a caregiver must take note regarding the development of cerebral palsy on a baby/child?

25. Provide five causes of birth defects.

26. What is a Down Syndrome?

27. Define amputation.

28. Give six examples of amputations.

29. What can be necessary devices can be provided to a person whose both hands are amputated?

30. What is mental retardation?

31. How can a caregiver note of mental retardation in a child?

32. How different is a mildly retarded person from a severely retarded person?

33. Is there a cure for mental retardation?

34. Aside from mental retardation, name five other mental impairments.

35. Differentiate fits from epilepsy.

# MODULE

## 6

### Preparation for Future Employment as a Caregiver

**MODULE 6**

MODULE 6
**SPECIAL PROJECT: MY FUTURE EMPLOYMENT**
**Total Allotted Time: 120 Hours**

TERMINAL OBJECTIVE OF MODULE 6:

Upon completion of Module 6, the participant will be able to:

- Have a thorough understanding of the community he or she will be living in.
- Describe in details and sketch the house of his or her future employer.
- Have a proposed or recommended Schedule of House Chores based on input from employer detailing daily, weekly and monthly chores.
- Provide a Month's Menu outlining Breakfast, Lunch , Supper including snacks.
- Have a complete profile of the person requiring care and a brief profile of the person's significant others.
- Provide a suggested Plan of Schedule of Activities
  For a child or children: Activities would reflect ages and stages of development
  For Persons with Special Needs: Activities would reflect SPICE capabilities.
- FOR PERSON WITH DISABILITY ONLY. Provide a review of literature on the ailments or disabilities of the person requiring care.
- Have a thorough understanding of the Rights and Freedom of the Caregiver while at work and on days off.
- Have a thorough understanding of the Live-in Caregiver Program and the caregiver's roles and legal responsibilities.

**MODULE 6 TOPIC OUTLINE**

| TOPICS | SUB-TOPICS |
|---|---|
| 6.1 My Canadian Community<br>(18 hours) | 6.1.1 The Community<br>6.1.2 The Nearest City<br>6.1.3 The Province |
| 2.2 My Home in Canada<br>(18 hours) | 6.2.1 The Structure of the Home<br>2.2.2 The Appliances in the Home<br>2.2.3 Proposed Schedule of House Chores |
| 3.4 Menu Planning<br>(18 hours) | 3.4.1 The Family's Favourites<br>3.4.2 Proposed Menu for the Month<br>3.4.3 Recipes in Index Cards |
| 4.7 The Person I Will Care For<br>(18 hours) | 4.7.1 The Profile of the Person Requiring Care<br>4.7.2 SPICE Characteristics<br>4.7.3 Schedule of Special Needs/Activities<br>4.7.4 *Current Literature on Disability<br>[For Special Need Person Caregiver] |
| 4.8 The Caregiver Rights/Freedom<br>(18 hours) | 6.5.1 Review of Canada's Rights & Freedom<br>6.5.2 The Labor Laws of Canada<br>6.5.3The Provincial Labor Standards (Canada)<br>6.5.4 My Days Off |
| 4.9 The Live-in Caregiver Program<br>(18 hours) | 6.6.1 Questions and Answers |

*The above lessons will thoroughly familiarize the trainee with his or her future employer.

Attempts should be made to regularly contact the employer through letters

# CONTENTS OF MODULE 6

# 6.1                     CANADA

## 6.1.1   A BRIEF HISTORY OF CANADA

Canada is the largest trading partner of the U.S. Unlike the U.S., Canada did not declare "independence" from Britain. Canada was declared a Dominion of Britain and was given its own constitution under the British North American Act of 1867.

July 1 is celebrated as the birth date of the Canadian constitution which took place in 1867. This new constitution allowed Canada to function without the interference of the British Parliament. Ontario, Quebec, New Brunswick and Nova Scotia made up the original Dominion of Canada.

Now, there are 10 provinces and 3 territories that comprise the country of Canada and are protected under the Canadian Constitution. Initially called Dominion Day, it was changed to Canada Day in 1982 to reflect the multicultural fabric of the country. Canada still has close ties to the United Kingdom, but is completely independent of British rule, enjoying the same status as other former commonwealth countries such as Australia and New Zealand.

Until one of the first known European explorers to land in Canada in 95 AD. Leif Ericson, a Viking settled in Newfoundland, nothing much was recorded in the history books of Canada. John Cabot (1497) under King Henry VII of England, Jacque Cartier (1534) under King Francis I of France, Samuel de Chaplain were some explorers who were recorded in Canadian history. They paved the way for the bloody exploration between the French and the British of the Great Lakes and the St. Lawrence waterway. The dispute known as the Seven Years War (1756-1763) between the French and English over North America concluded in 1763.

## 6.1.2   NATIONAL ANTHEM

### 6-1
### <u>O'CANADA</u>

| | |
|---|---|
| O Canada | O Canada |
| Our home and native land | We stand on guard on thee |
| True patriot love | God keep our land |
| In all our sons command | Glorious and free |
| With glowing hearts | O Canada we stand on guard for thee |
| We see thee rise | O Canada we stand on guard for thee |
| Our true north strong and free | |

## 6.1.3  GENERAL GEOGRAPHY

### 6-2

❖ Canada is an independent nation.

❖ Second largest country in the world (3,831,012 sq. mi/9,922.330 sq.km).

❖ It comprises 10 provinces and 3 Federal Territories.

❖ The Prairie Provinces:
ALBERTA
MANITOBA
SASKATCHEWAN

❖ The Atlantic Provinces: NEW BRUNSWICK
NOVA SCOTIA
PRINCE EDWARD  ISLAND
NEWFOUNDLAND
(The first three are also known as the Maritime Provinces)

❖ QUEBEC is known as Francophone (French Speaking) Province, ONTARIO, and BRITISH COLUMBIA.

❖ The territories:          YUKON
NUNAVUT
NORTHWEST TERRITORIES

❖ The capital of Canada is the OTTAWA.

❖ Provincial Capitals:

| | | |
|---|---|---|
| British Columbia (BC) | - | **Victoria** |
| Alberta (AB) | - | **Edmonton** |
| Saskatchewan (Sask) | - | **Regina** |
| Manitoba(Man) | - | **Winnipeg** |
| Ontario (Ont) | - | **Toronto** |
| Quebec (Que) | - | **Quebec** |
| Prince Edward Island (P.E.I) | - | **Charlottetown** |
| New Brunswick (NB) | - | **Fredericton** |
| Nova Scotia (NS) | - | **Halifax** |
| Yukon Territories(YT) | - | **Whitehorse** |
| Northwest Territories (NT or NWT) | - | **Yellowknife** |
| Nunavut | - | **Iqaluit** |
| Newfoundland (NFL) | - | **St. John's** |

## 6.1.4  FACTS AND FIGURES

(Reprinted from http://geodepot.statcan.ca/Diss/Highlights/Page1/Page1_
e.cfm)

### *2001 Canada Population Census*

Canada has experienced one of the smallest census-to-census growth rates in its population. Between 1996 and 2001, the nation's population increased by 1,160,333 people, a gain of 4%. The Census counted 30,007,094 people in Canada on May 15, 2001, compared with 28,846,761 in 1996. Growth rates decelerated in every province except Alberta, compared with the early 1990s.

Only three provinces and one territory registered growth rates above the national average of 4%. Alberta's population surged by 10.3%, compared with 5.9% between 1991 and 1996. Ontario gained 6.1%, British Columbia 4.9% and Nunavut 8.1%.

Six provinces experienced small changes in population (less than 1.5% in either direction): Prince Edward Island, Nova Scotia, New Brunswick, Quebec, Manitoba and Saskatchewan.

The population of Newfoundland and Labrador declined for the second consecutive census period. Between 1996 and 2001, the province's population decreased 7%, more than double the 2.9% rate of decline during the previous five years. Yukon Territory and the Northwest Territories also showed declines of more than 5%.

For Canada as a whole, immigration was the main source of growth in population between 1996 and 2001, as the nation experienced a decline of about one-third in natural increase (the difference between births and deaths) compared with the previous 5-year period.

The trend in urbanization continued. In 2001, 79.4% of Canadians lived in an urban area with a population of 10,000 people or more, compared with 78.5% in 1996.

Seven of 27 census metropolitan areas had a growth rate at least double that of the national average of 4%; the largest growth rates were in Calgary, Oshawa and Toronto.

From 1996 to 2001, the nation's population has continued to concentrate further in four broad urban regions: the extended Golden Horseshoe in southern Ontario; Montréal and its adjacent region; the Lower Mainland of British Columbia and southern Vancouver Island; and the Calgary-Edmonton corridor[1]. Between 1996 and 2001, these four regions combined grew 7.6% compared with virtually no growth (+0.5%) in the rest of the country. In 2001, 51% of Canada's population lived in these regions compared with

| | | |
|---|---|---|
| **People.** | Population (1992 est): | 27,351,000 |
| | Age distribution (%): | 0-14     20.9 |
| | | 15-59    63.1 |
| | | 60 +     16.0 |

**Pop density.**   7 per sq. mi, Urban (1990)       77%

| **Ethnic groups.** | British | 25% |
|---|---|---|
| | French | 24% |
| | Other European | 16% |
| | Mixed | 28% |

**Language.**          English, French (both official)

| **Religion.** | Roman Catholic | 46% |
|---|---|---|
| | Protestant | 41% |

**Geography.**      Area, 3,849,672 sq. mi., the largest country in land size in the western hemisphere. Canada stretches 3,426 miles from east to west and extended southward from the North pole to the US border. Its seacoast included 36,356 miles of mainland and 115,113 miles of islands, including the Arctic islands almost from Greenland to near the Alaskan border.

**Climate.**        While generally temperate, varies from freezing winter cold to blistering summer heat.

**Capital.**         Ottawa.

| Cities (met.2001 est): | |
|---|---|
| Montreal | 3,426,350 |
| Vancouver | 1,986, 965 |
| Ottawa-Hull | 1,063,664 |
| Winnipeg | 671,274 |
| Edmonton | 937,845 |
| Calgary | 951,395 |
| Quebec | 682,757 |
| Toronto | 4,682, 897 |

**Finance.**        Monetary unit: dollar (May 2003: CDN$1.39= US $1)

**Transport.**      Railroads (1990):    Length:           56,771 mi.
                     Motor vehicles: in use (1989):      12.0 million
                     Passenger cars:                 3.7 million
                     Comm. Civil Aviation (1990):   46 billion
                     Passenger – km: 106 airports with scheduled       flights.

**Local Divisions.**      10 Provinces and 3 Territories

| **Communications.** | Television sets: | 1 per 1.7 persons |
| | Radios: | 1 per 1.2 persons |
| | Telephones in use: | 1 per 1.3 persons |
| | Daily newspaper circa (1991): | 187 per 1,000 pop. |

| **Health.** | Life expectancy at birth | |
| | 1992: | 74 male, 81 female |
| | Births (per 1,000 pop.1992): | 14 |

| **Deaths:** | (per 1,000 pop 1992): | 7 |
| | Natural increase: | 7% |
| | Hospital beds: | 1 per 148 persons |

**Physicians.**    1 per 449 persons.
Infant mortality (per 1,000 live birth 1992): 7.3

| **Education.** | (1991): Literacy: | 99% |

**Major International Organizations.** UN and all of its specialized agencies, NATO, OECD.

**Commonwealth of Nations.** Canada became the first nation to ratify the North American Free Trade Agreement between Canada, Mexico and the US on June 23, 1993.

## 6.1.5  Canadian Government

Canada's government is modeled after a Confederation with Parliamentary Democracy. There are two levels of government: Canada (bicameral) the Provincial and the Federal Government.

The head of state of Canada is her Majesty, Queen Elizabeth II who is represented by the Governor General at the Federal level and the Lieutenant Governor at the Provincial level.

At the Federal level, the head of the government is known the Prime Minister. The Prime Minister is not voted into office but is the leader of the party with the most seats in the House of Commons.

At the Provincial level, the head of the government is known as the Premier. Like the Prime Minister, the Premier is not voted in but is the leader of the party with the majority of the seats in the Legislative Assembly.

## 6.1.6  Regions of Canada

The provinces Alberta, Manitoba & Saskatchewan, collectively known  as  the Prairie Provinces New Brunswick, Nova Scotia, Prince Edward  Island and Newfoundland known as Atlantic Provinces (The first three also being called the Maritime Provinces),  QUEBEC is known as Francophone (French Speaking) Province, Ontario, and British Columbia. The territories are the Yukon, Nunavut and the Northwest Territories.

## 6.2                                                  LIFE IN CANADA

*Life is new country is not a bed of roses. Many problems of a newcomer stems from the need to cope with life in a new environment (physical, social, psychological and language).*

### 6.2.1   THE ACCULTURATION PROCESS

It is important to be aware that a newcomer both young and old, undergoes certain psychological stages in acculturating himself. Each of these stages may either be brief or lingering depending on the individual.

First, he goes through the **Tourist Stage**. Everything is new, exciting, fascinating and the people around are friendly, hospitable, understanding and sympathetic. He usually feels very good and very positive about himself. Days are long or prolonged as he visits new acquaintances and places.

Eventually, he goes through the **Homesick Stage**. In this stage he misses his motherland, his families or relatives, his friends and most of all his old way of life. Letters and phone calls do not seem enough to relieve the aching feeling that he experiences.

This stage is followed by the **Decision Stage**. He must decide whether to stay in the new country, go back home or move to a new location.

Then comes the **Rooting or Settling Stage**. The newcomer has decided to stay. He is now ready to adopt the new country, adapt his ways and become an immigrant. He is now ready to make roots and can now begin the long process of building his own identity in his adopted land. He becomes a visitor to his mother country. To those who succeed and adopt the new country, the acculturation is complete and smooth. To those who failed to integrate and acculturate, the process becomes incomplete and the newcomer becomes an outsider, never knowing how to adapt and acculturate. By realizing the above stages a newcomer may become better prepared on what to expect.

### *Stages of Acculturation*

### Stage 1 – The Tourist Stage

> When a newcomer arrives in a new country, he has a feeling of well being and excitement. He is in many ways a tourist. Everything around him seems new, clean and modern. The people around him are friendly, generous and hospitable. Although tired from his trip, he feels like exploring the new surroundings – in fact, the new environment (physical, social, and cultural). His unspoken questions may consist of the following:

> 1.    What is really here?
> 2.    How big is this community? This city?
> 3.    What familiar things are here?

4.  How many people are here from my country? Where are they?
5.  Where I am going to live? What are the choices?
6.  Will I have a neighbor from my own country that I can meet?
7.  Is there a group or organization from my country that I can meet?
8.  Where I can go for help?
9.  Do they speak my language?
10. Is there an interpreter I can count on?
11. Where is my money going to come from? How am I going to budget it?
12. What are my priorities?
13. What happens when I get sick?
14. What kind of food am I going to eat?
15. Where can I get my kind of food?
16. Where do I go to mail my postcard? A letter? A parcel?
17. I'm married and have children. Where will the children go to school?
18. How different schools are here? What grade level will my children be? Will they repeat (a) grades(s)?
19. What is my spouse going to do?
20. Where can I get a camera? Where can I get films developed?
21. How expensive are long distance calls?
22. How long does it take to get letter to my country?

## Stage 2 – The Homesick Stage

➢ Depending on the personality of the newcomer and how the community receives him, he may linger in this stage (from a few weeks to even years). Any one stage may overlap with the rest of the acculturation stages.

➢ The newcomer will attempt to adapt and will try some of his old ways and means (habit). As a result three factors may affect the newcomer:

♦ The new society or community requires certain expected behavior and the newcomer may or may not be able to meet the expectation.

♦ The new society or community may not accept the newcomer's behavior and he, therefore, becomes unprepared for society's reaction. He may exhibit confusion, submission, eagerness to learn or may become unresponsive and uncooperative. He may also experience total acceptance and become very comfortable in the community's way of life.

♦ The community's behavior may totally be unacceptable to the newcomer. This may lead to conflict and a total readjustment altogether.

### *During the homesick stage questions may consist of:*

1.  I wonder what my relatives or friends are doing now?
2.  I wonder who is looking after our properties?

3. Will I ever see my country again?
4. If I call, I wonder who will answer the phone? Will they all be home at this time?
5. I wonder what time it is over there? Is it daytime? Nighttime?
6. I wonder if they are missing me (us) right now?
7. I wonder who has some music from my country? Where can I buy them?
8. Are there movies from my country here? How often are they showing? Where do I go to rent them?
9. Will I ever see my country again?  my friends?

## Stage 3 – Realization or Confrontation Stage

> The newcomer begins to see the difference between his culture and the new way of life here. He begins to accept and reject expectations. He begins to questions his identity, his self-worth. He begins to question his status quo. He starts looking for alternatives. He begins to look at his future. When he begins to question his old habits or ways and means, unconsciously he will keep those that he thinks will enhance his culture and reject those that seem not appropriate or acceptable to him.

### *Questions or comments during this stage may consist of:*

1. I wonder if I should attend ESL classes?
2. Boy, is he ever dumb?
3. Should I let them know I know how to do the job?
4. Gosh, I am overqualified for this job!
5. Where can I find another job?
6. Will I be able to change jobs without going broke.
7. I can't give you my leftover medicine. Should you not really go to a doctor instead?
8. I wonder if I'll ever make it here. I feel dumb sometimes.
9. It's so frustrating not to join in their conversation!
10. They think they are so smart!

## Stage 4 – Decision Stage
> The newcomer has to make some decision.
1. His job-what kind?
2. What training?
3. Are his qualifications adequate?
4. Can he find a job with his training and qualifications?
5. What are the alternatives?
6. How does he find out?
7. Where does he look? What does he need?
8. What about his pay? Is one job enough?
9. Sources of funds?
10. Re-training? Improvement courses?
11. Should he go back to his old country?
12. Should he stay? Racial prejudice? Discrimination?
13. What about a trip home? A short visit?

14. His new friends? How active should he be in the community?
15. Climate? Too cold? Can he adjust?
16. Spouse happy? Children adjusting well?

## Stage 5 – Settlement (Rooting) Stage

➤ Psychologically, the newcomer is ready to settle down. He has decided to stay. What are his long range plans for himself? His family?

➤ He has accepted the new society. He is now ready to become an economically independent individual. He is ready to extend help to others. He can now prepare himself in becoming a true North American. He has to prepare for his citizenship.

➤ He is now a productive member of his community. He can volunteer some of his time and contribute some of his knowledge base and life experience.

### *Comments may consist of:*

1. Where can I find information regarding a house?
2. I better start saving!
3. How do I find out about the requirements of becoming a citizen?
4. I would like to sit on your Board of Directors!
5. I guess I can volunteer as an interpreter twice a week.
6. The university syllabus finally came!
7. What are my rights as a Canadian?
8. I should really look for a part-time job in addition to my full time employment.

## *The Old vs. The New Way of Life*

➤ The newcomer's thoughts and feelings, indeed his whole identity and personality were formed and shaped by his old way of life which, in some significant cases is different from the new way of life. One of the stumbling blocks is the new everyday language. Through his first language, he developed his own personality and handled his life experiences. In his new environment (North America), he is now faced with the problems of dealing with similar life experiences but by means of translated words and sentences. But the point is, he sees, feels, hears as he does largely because of his language habits developed in his first language. The tragedy of the situation is that his first language, which is an integral part of his personality, now stands in the way of acquiring and even mastering a new language, a new way of life, a new life.

➤ Depending on what part of the old country a newcomer comes from, his way of life may conflict with the assertive, competitive, materialistic and independent way of life of North Americans.

### *Loss of Prestige and Status*

> ➢ Newcomers often experience a loss of face, status and prestige. They find many situations difficult to cope with.

> ➢ In their own countries, they may have been successful or respected in business and the professions. They now have to accept what the old way of life or "culture" considers menial or degrading work because they cannot meet the new professional requirements- almost always this includes the mastery of English.

> ➢ Even when the new language learner has acquired fluent English, the fact that he has an accent or his color is different tends to imply that he does not completely belong. "Gee, I though you were born here, your English is very good!" " Where are you from, you have adapted very well!"

> ➢ The chief problem facing the newcomer is psychological and emotional in nature. He has an excess of self-consciousness. He is overly conscious of the way he speaks and sounds out new words. Therefore, he may prefer to stay away from meetings, social gatherings or events that will force him to enter into any kind of conversation or discussion-the very activities that would speed his language acquisition and integration into the mainstream of North American life. He is terrified of appearing foolish and knows that his first faltering steps in English are the object or ridicule, if anything. He must also be actually immersed and exercised in the behavior patterns of the English language community if he is to learn to orally communicate with any depth. In a sense, the humor or ridicule produced by faulty pronunciation and/or sentence construction is a necessary reinforcement in the stages of language acquisition.

"My pronunciation teacher (my late husband) used the "ridicule" approach (he would laughed when he corrected my pronunciation) when my tongue slipped back to my old oral habits. Then he would swear that I had no sense of humor when I refused to even talk to him for days." The thing to remember is, many times, in trying to help, the means do not justify the end. Hence, most new language learners shun situations where they may appear foolish and sacrifice opportunities for practice but they are the only way to orally become fluent. (language immersion). My late husband had this to say by the way. "I do not intend to ridicule my wife when I correct her. But please understand, I do not know how to deal with it myself. All I know is I must help her overcome her apparent problems. I sometimes feel embarrassed myself in correcting her that I unconsciously laugh, I think, to hide my uncomfortable feeling." (Bless his soul and may he rest in peace. I miss him so much!)

> ➢ Mixed attitudes towards North American way of life may lead to confusion. Individuality and independence are encouraged here and the newcomer may interpret this as a "DO AS YOU PLEASE" culture. However, they cannot get over the fact that this same culture has strict and authoritative rules on child, adult and drug abuse.

**To the Newcomer...**

As a newcomer, you have made great sacrifices in coming to North America. Canada, after all, has been built upon generations of immigrants whose greatest desire has been to be a Canadian. Canada is a land of opportunity-respect her, build her up and once you have your immigrant/Canadian status, enjoy Canada's Charter of Rights and Freedoms.

## 6.3 CAREGIVER'S RIGHTS AND RESPONSIBILITIES

### 6.3.1 PROVINCIAL LABOR STANDARDS

> Labor standards is a matter dealt at the Provincial Level of the Canadian Governing Body. As such, each province has its own standards of labor which vary slightly but all deal with the protection of the employee and in some ways the employer as well. Below is a list of contact WebPages for each province and territory.

| | |
|---|---|
| British Columbia: | http://www.labour.gov.bc.ca/esb/ |
| Alberta: | http://www.gov.ab.ca/home/ |
| Saskatchewan: | http://www.labour.gov.sk.ca/standards/index.htm |
| Manitoba: | http://www.gov.mb.ca/labour/standards/index.html |
| Ontario: | http://www.gov.on.ca/lab/english/es/index.html |
| Quebec: | http://www.cnt.gouv.qc.ca/en/index.asp |
| Newfoundland: | http://www.gov.nf.ca/labour/ |
| Nova Scotia: | http://www.gov.ns.ca/enla/labrstd.htm |
| New Brunswick: | http://www.gov.nb.ca/0308/0001e.htm |
| Nunavut: | http://www.gov.nu.ca/ |
| Northwest Territories: | http://www.gov.nt.ca/ |
| Yukon Territories: | http://www.gov.yk.ca/depts/community/labour/ |
| | |
| CANADA: | http://www.gov.cic.ca |

### Employment Standards

> Employment Standards mandate the minimum standards of employment for employers and employees in the work place. Through the Employment Standards Code and the Standards Regulation, they let the employer and employee to be informed of what is acceptable labor practices in each province. Examples are issues such as payment of earnings, hours of work, rest periods, and day of rest, overtime and overtime pay, general holidays and vacation pay, maternal and paternal leave, termination of employment, and employment for individuals under the age of 18. For live-in caregivers, Labor Standards can only interfere on matters that are covered in the Employer-Employee contract, therefore it is crucial that a caregiver has an updated written Contract of Employment.

### Complaint Resolution Process

1. File a formal written letter of complaint to a Provincial Labor Officer. When the Labor Officer approves your case the employer is notified and a copy of the letter is sent to the employer and requests a review of the issue.

2. If the employer responds and the issue is dealt with, the complaint is settled.

3. If the employee feels that issues aren't fully settled as agreed upon by the employer and the employee, documentation proof must be sent to the Labor Officer handling the case.

4. Officer investigates further as necessary.

## 6.3.2  THE CANADIAN CHARTER OF RIGHTS AND FREEDOMS

| Rights and Freedoms | What You Can Do |
|---|---|
| **Fundamental Freedoms** | - worship as you like<br>- believe what you want<br>- express your opinions<br>- associate with whomever you like<br>- gather together peacefully |
| **Democratic Rights** | - vote in elections<br>- run as a candidate in elections<br>- elect a government at least every 3-5 years |
| **Mobility Rights** | - enter, remain in, or leave Canada |
| **Legal Rights** | - enjoy life, liberty and security of a person have a fair trial if accused of a crime |
| **Equality Rights** | - live and work and be protected by the law without discrimination based on race, national or ethnic origin, color, religion sex, age, or mental or physical disability |
| **Language Rights** | - communicate with, and receive available services from any federal government office in either French or English<br>- use either English or French in any court<br>- have your children educated in either English or French |
| **Enforcement** | - take the matter to court if any of the above rights and freedoms have been denied |
| **General** | - Native people retain their rights<br>- the charter should be interpreted to enhance Canada's multi cultural heritage<br><br>- the charter applies equally to males and females<br>- references in the Charter to provinces also includes territories |

## 6.3.3  HUMAN RIGHTS, CITIZENSHIP AND MULTICULTURALISM ACT OF 1996

The Individual's Rights Protection Act of 1972 was created to protect visible minorities from discrimination.  The underlying principles of the Act states that,  with regards to a person's race, religious beliefs, color, gender, physical disability, mental disability, ancestry, place of origin, marital status, source of income or family status of that person or class of person of any other person or class of persons share in the same rights as follows:

> ➢ All peoples are equal.

> ➢ No person may deny any goods, services, accommodation or facilities that are customarily available to the general public.

> ➢ No person shall be allowed to publicly issue or display publications, notices, signs, symbols, emblems, or other representation that has the intent to discriminate other persons or to incite hatred against any person or group.

> ➢ An employer does not have the right to refuse employment, terminate employment, or discriminate an employee on the basis of race, religious beliefs, color, gender, physical disability, mental disability, ancestry, place of origin, marital status, source of income or family status of that person or class of person of any other person or class of persons.

> ➢ If an employee is paid less than the agreed rate with the employer, the employee has the right to claim the difference within 12 months of the cause of action.

| 6.4 | THE CAREGIVER'S APPLICATION FOR TEMPORARY RESIDENT VISA |
|---|---|

### 6.4.1  The Process of Application at HRCC

> ➤ Once you have secured a prospective employer, the employer will send a request letter to hire you to the HRCC. The HRCC (Human Resources Center Canada) will check whether there is no available Canadian workers (advertisements at a major newspaper must accompany the application) to fill the position and will send a letter back to your prospective employer. If the request is approved, the employer will send you a copy of the approval letter. The approval letter allows you to submit a formal application for a working Visa in Canada.

> ➤ The application form for a working Visa will require you to send proof of education papers (i.e. diplomas, transcript of records) and proof of experience. You may also be required to go through an interview with a Visa officer. An incomplete application form will forfeit your application.

> ➤ Upon the approval of your application form, you will be required to have a medical test and apply for a passport and a Temporary Resident Visa.

### 6.4.2  THE JOB OFFER AND EMPLOYER-EMPLOYEE CONTRACT

> ➤ After the job offer has been made and both employer and employee have agreed to such an arrangement, the employer must fill out the LIVE-IN CAREGIVER PROGRAM Information Guide which is stated previously before getting confirmation from the CIC. Within the Information Guide is a sample Live-In Caregiver Contract.

> ➤ The contract is a written agreement between you and your employer on the terms of employment. It is there to clarify any misunderstandings on the terms of employment and as a reference to authorities when labor and employment standards have been violated. See samples of contract below.

### 6.4.3  REQUIRED DOCUMENTS

Below is a list of required documents for the application process.

- A copy of the Confirmation of Job Offer Letter
- Working Visa Application
- School Transcripts, Diplomas, or proof of experience documents, and proof of training documents
- Passport
- Temporary Resident  Visa
- Working Visa

## 6.4.4  THE APPLICATION KIT

The following 4 pages are samples of the Application Kit you are required to fill out.

## Child Care Sample Contract

### *LIVE-IN CAREGIVER CONTRACT*

1. Employer
   Name: _____
   Address: _____
   Telephone: Home ( ) _____
            Work ( ) _____

   Revenue Canada Employer Number

2. Employee
   Name: _____
   Address: _____

3. Offer of Employment

   Job Title: Live-in Caregiver

A) Job Description:

Child Care   Yes _____ No _____   Number of Children _____   Ages of Children:_____
Housekeeping Responsibilies   Yes _____ No _____
Describe _____
_____

Will employee be required to provide pet care?   Yes _____   No _____
Additional Responsiblities   Yes _____   No _____
Description of the House and Household (number of rooms, household members ) _____

B) Wages and Working Conditions

Wages and working conditions must reflect provincial employment standards and prevailing wages rates.

Gross Wage of $ _____ _____ Weekly   Hours of Work ____/wk   Frequency of Pay _____ weekly
                    _____ Monthly   Number of Days off ____/wk        _____ biweekly
                             List Days off _____           _____ monthly
Overtime Rate $ _____/hr   To be paid after ____ hours/day _____ hours/week
Schedule of Hours _____

The employer agrees to provide the employee with the information regarding wages and types and approximate values of all deduction from wages.

Number of weeks Vacation with Pay _____     Paid General Holidays _____
Other types of Leave _____     Number of sick days/year _____

Cost of Room and Board $ _____   To be paid _____ weekly _____ monthly
Accommodation: Furnished Private Room Yes __ No __ Locked Yes __ No__ Private Bath Yes __No__

Medical Coverage: _____
Airfare Included   Yes _____ No _____
Details _____

_____ Income tax Deductions will be taken at source.
_____ Contribution will be made by employer to Canada/Quebec Pension Plan and to Unemployment insurance
Duration of Employment: _____

4) Terms of Separation
The employer and the Employee agrees to abide by provincial labour standards regarding written notice of termination of employment. (It is recommended that a copy of the relevant portions of provincial labour standards be attached as an appendix.) Amendments to this contract must be made in writing and agreed to by both parties.

5) Signature of Employer
I certify that the duties outlined above are accurate and correct. I will abide by provincial standards. I will provide a Record of Employment on Termination of Employment.

Signature _____     Date _____

6) Signature of Employee
I have read the undertaking and understand it

Signature _____     Date _____

## **Elderly Care Sample Contract**

### *LIVE-IN CAREGIVER CONTRACT*

1.  Employer
    Name: _____
    Address: _____
    Telephone: Home ( ) _____
                 Work ( ) _____

    Revenue Canada Employer Number

2.  Employee
    Name: _____
    Address: _____

3.  Offer of Employment

    Job Title:  Live-in Caregiver

A)  Job Description:

Elderly Care   Yes ____ No _____    Disabled Care  Yes _____ No _____
Housekeeping Responsibilies   Yes _____ No _____
Describe _____

_____
_____

Will employee be required to provide pet care?  Yes ____ No ____
Additional Responsiblities  Yes ____ No ____
Description of the House and Household (number of rooms, household members ) _____

B)  Wages and Working Conditions

Wages and working conditions must refect provincial employment standards and prevailing wages rates.

Gross Wage of $ _____ ___   Weekly   Hours of Work _____ /wk   Frequency of Pay _____   weekly
                  ___ Monthly   Number of Days off ____ /wk               _____ biweekly
                                  List Days off _____                        _____ monthly
Overtime Rate $ _____ /hr   To be paid after _____ hours/day   _____ hours/week
Schedule of Hours _____

The employer agrees to provide the employee with the information regarding wages and types and approximate values of all deduction from wages.

Number of weeks Vacation with Pay _____    Paid General Holidays _____
Other types of Leave _____    Number of sick days/year _____

Cost of Room and Board $ _____ To be paid _____ weekly _____ monthly
Accommodation:  Furnished Private Room  Yes __ No __ Locked  Yes __ No__ Private Bath Yes __ No__

Medical Coverage: _____
Airfare Included  Yes _____ No _____
Details _____

____ Income tax Deductions will be taken at source.
____ Contribution will be made by employer to Canada/Quebec Pension Plan and to Unemployment insurance
Duration of Employment: _____

4)  Terms of Separation
    The employer and the Employee agrees to abide by provincial labour standards regarding written notice of termination of employment. (It is recommended that a copy of the relevant portions of provincial labour standards be attached as an appendix.) Amendments to this contract must be made in writing and agreed to by both parties.

5)  Signaure of Employer
    I certify that the duties outlined above are accurate and correct. I will abide by provincial standards. I will provide a Record of Employment on Termination of Employment.

    Signature _____    Date _____

6)  Signature of Employee
    I have read the undertaking and understand it

    Signature _____    Date _____

Canadian Embassy             Immigration Section          Ambassade du Canada
9<sup>th</sup> Floor, Allied Bank Centre                          MAILING ADDRESS
6754 Ayala Avenue                                        P.O. Box 2098 MCPO
Makati, Metro Manila         Fax (632) 810-4659          Makati, Metro Manila

### APPLICATION FOR A WORK PERMIT AS A LIVE-IN CAREGIVER

PLEASE SUBMIT YOUR APPLICATION BY MAIL OR IN PERSON TO THE DROP BOX IN THE EMBASSY LOBBY. DO NOT SUBMIT YOUR APPLICATION UNLESS IT IS COMPLETED FULLY AND YOU HAVE ALL THE REQUIRED DOCUMENTS. AN APPLICATION THAT IS INCOMPLETE WILL BE RETURNED TO YOU.

TO ASSIST US IN ASSESSING YOUR APPLICATION, PLEASE SUBMIT THE FOLLOWING:

- NON-REFUNDABLE processing fee of Ca$150 or PhP4,800.
  Fees MUST be paid by **MANAGER'S CHEQUE, CERTIFIED CHEQUE, POSTAL MONEY ORDER or BANK DRAFT** payable to the "Canadian Embassy, Manila". Cash will **NOT** be accepted.
- Completed Application for a Work Permit (attached)
- Completed Family Composition Form (attached)
- Completed Education and Work History Form (attached)
- Four (4) recent passport-sized photographs
- A recent NBI clearance marked "**Visa-Canada**"
- Original records of your education after high school, including Transcript of Records,
- Proof of successful completion of at least six months of full-time training in a classroom setting in a field or occupation related to the job offered in Canada. OR One year of full-time paid employment within the last three years, including at least six months of continuous employment with one employer in a job related to the prospective employment in Canada.
- Letters of reference from present or past employers which detail your duties.

> **NOTE:**
> ALL DOCUMENTS
> MUST BE ORIGINAL

Completion of the forms and payment of the processing fee **do not** guarantee acceptance of your application. Once we have received and reviewed your submission, we will advise you further in writing concerning a personal interview or other requirements which may apply. If you do not hear from us within 90 days you may follow-up in writing or by fax. Please do not enquire before the 90 days have expired, your request will not be answered. Due to Canadian privacy laws, we can not give any information over the telephone.

Additional information on Canada's Live-in Caregiver Program may be found on the internet at the following site: www.cic.gc.ca/english/visit/caregi_e.html

**NOTE : You will be required to undergo and pass at your own expense a prescribed medical examination. Medical examination forms will be given to you at your interview.**

lcp-Info-req-irpa (06/02)

**Citizenship and Immigration Canada** / **Citoyenneté et Immigration Canada**

# APPLICATION FOR A WORK PERMIT
# DEMANDE D'UN PERMIS DE TRAVAIL

I want service in:
Je veux être servi(e) en :
☐ English / Anglais    ☐ French / Français

File - Référence

**1** Surname (Family name) · Nom de famille | First name - Prénom | Middle name - Autre(s) prénom(s)

**2** My current mailing address. All correspondence will go to this address. If you wish to authorize the release of information from your case file to a representative, indicate their address below and on the form IMM 5476.
Mon adresse postale actuelle. Toute la correspondance sera envoyée à cette adresse. Si vous désirez autoriser la transmission de renseignements ou ouvrant votre dossier à un représentant, indiquez son adresse ci-dessous et sur le formulaire IMM 5476.

**3** My residential address (if different from your mailing address)
Mon adresse personnelle (si elle est différente de votre adresse postale)

Telephone number ► | Fax number ►
Numéro de téléphone | Numéro de télécopieur

**4** Date of birth-Date de naissance    D-J  M  Y-A

**5** Place of birth - Lieu de naissance
City/Town - Ville/Village | Prov./State - Prov./État | Country - Pays

**6** Citizen of - Citoyenneté

**7** Sex - Sexe
☐ Male / Homme    ☐ Female / Femme

**8** Present marital status - État civil
☐ Unmarried (never married) / Célibataire  ☐ Engaged / Fiancé(e)  ☐ Married / Marié(e)  ☐ Widowed / Veuf (Veuve)  ☐ Separated / Séparé(e)  ☐ Divorced / Divorcé(e)  ☐ Common law / Conjoint de fait

**9** Personal details of family members (spouse or common-law partner and dependent children)
Renseignements sur les membres de ma famille (conjoint(e) ou conjoint(e) de fait et enfants dépendants)

| | APPLICANT REQUÉRANT | SPOUSE OR COMMON-LAW PARTNER AND CHILDREN ÉPOUX OU CONJOINT DE FAIT ET ENFANTS | | |
|---|---|---|---|---|
| Family name / Nom de famille | | | | |
| First and second names / Prénom(s) | | | | |
| Relationship / Lien de parenté | SELF LUI-MÊME | | | |
| Date of birth / Date de naissance | D-J M Y-A | D-J M Y-A | D-J M Y-A | D-J M Y-A |
| Place of birth / Lieu de naissance | | | | |
| Citizenship / Citoyenneté | | | | |
| Passport no. / N° de passeport | | | | |
| Passport expiry date / Date d'expiration du passeport | D-J M Y-A | D-J M Y-A | D-J M Y-A | D-J M Y-A |
| Marital status / État matrimonial | | | | |
| Will accompany you to Canada? Vous accompagnera au Canada? | | ☐ Yes/Oui ☐ No/Non | ☐ Yes/Oui ☐ No/Non | ☐ Yes/Oui ☐ No/Non |

**10**

**DO NOT WRITE IN THIS SPACE**
**ESPACE RÉSERVÉ**

Officer - Agent

THIS FORM HAS BEEN ESTABLISHED BY THE MINISTER OF CITIZENSHIP AND IMMIGRATION
FORMULAIRE ÉTABLI PAR LE MINISTRE DE LA CITOYENNETÉ ET DE L'IMMIGRATION

IMM 1295 (06-2002) B

**Canada**

| 11 | My present job is (Give your job title and a brief description of your position) Profession actuelle (Indiquer le titre de votre emploi et une brève description du poste) | 12 | I have held my present job for J'occupe mon emploi actuel depuis | Month(s) Mois | Year(s) An(s) |
|----|----|----|----|----|----|

| 13 | The name and address of my employer and the type of business are - Nom et adresse de mon employeur (préciser également le genre d'entreprise) |
|----|----|

| 14 | The name and address of my prospective employer in Canada are (Attach original offer of employment) Nom et adresse de mon employeur éventuel au Canada (Joindre l'original de l'offre d'emploi) |
|----|----|

| 15 | My occupation in Canada will be (Give your job title and a brief description of your position) Ma profession au Canada sera (Indiquer le titre de votre emploi et une brève description du poste) | 16 | My salary will be - Mon salaire sera de $ Cdn.    $ (Canadiens) |
|----|----|----|----|

| 17 | I am expected to start my employment on Je suis censé commencer à travailler le | ▶ | D - J   M   Y - A | 18 | My employment is expected to finish on Il est prévu que mon emploi prendra fin le | ▶ | D - J   M   Y - A |
|----|----|----|----|----|----|----|----|

| 19 | Have you or any member of your family ever: Les questions suivantes s'adressent également au visiteur et à tout membre de sa famille | ("X" the appropriate box) (Inscrire « X » dans la case appropriée) |
|----|----|----|

| | a) | Been treated for any serious physical or mental disorders or any communicable or chronic diseases? Vous a-t-on jamais traité(e) pour une maladie mentale ou physique grave, ou pour une maladie contagieuse ou chronique? | ☐ Yes Oui  ☐ No Non |
|--|--|--|--|
| | b) | Committed, been arrested or charged with any criminal offence in any country? Avez-vous commis, ou avez-vous été arrêté pour avoir commis une infraction pénale quelconque dans n'importe quel pays? | ☐ Yes Oui  ☐ No Non |
| | c) | Been refused admission to, or ordered to leave Canada? Vous a-t-on jamais refusé l'admission au Canada, ou enjoint de quitter le Canada? | ☐ Yes Oui  ☐ No Non |
| | d) | Applied for any Canadian immigration visas (e.g. Permanent Resident, Student, Worker, Temporary Resident (visitor), Temporary Resident Permit)? Avez-vous demandé un visa canadien auparavant? (par exemple, un visa de résident permanent, d'étudiant, de travailleur, de résident temporaire [visiteur] ou un permis de séjour temporaire)? | ☐ Yes Oui  ☐ No Non |
| | e) | Been refused a visa to travel to Canada? Vous a-t-on jamais refusé un visa pour le Canada? | ☐ Yes Oui  ☐ No Non |
| | f) | In periods of either peace or war, have you ever been involved in the commission of a war crime or crime against humanity, such as: willful killing, torture, attacks upon, enslavement, starvation or other inhumane acts committed against civilians or prisoners of war, or deportation of civilians? En période de paix ou de guerre, avez-vous déjà participé à la commission d'un crime de guerre ou d'un crime contre l'humanité, c'est-à-dire de tout acte inhumain commis contre des populations civiles ou des prisonniers de guerre, par exemple, l'assassinat, la torture, l'agression, la réduction en esclavage ou la privation de nourriture, etc., ou encore participé à la déportation de civils? | ☐ Yes Oui  ☐ No Non |

If the answer to any of the above is "yes", give details - Si vous avez répondu « oui » à l'une ou l'autre question ci-dessus, veuillez préciser

| 20 | During the past five years have you or any family member accompanying you lived in any other country than your country of citizenship or permanent residence for more than six months? Au cours des cinq dernières années, avez-vous ou n'importe quel membre de votre famille vous accompagnant a-t-il vécu dans un autre pays que votre pays de citoyenneté ou de résidence permanente pendant plus de six mois? | ▶ | ☐ Yes Oui  ☐ No Non |
|----|----|----|----|

| 21 | If answer to question 20 is "yes" list countries and length of stay Si la réponse à la question 20 est affirmative, indiquer le nom de ces pays et la durée du séjour |
|----|----|

| Name Nom | Country Pays | Length of stay - Durée du séjour |  |
|----|----|----|----|
| | | From - De  D - J   M   Y - A | To - À  D - J   M   Y - A |
| | | | |
| | | | |
| | | | |

| 22 | I declare that I have answered all required questions in this application fully and truthfully Je déclare avoir donné des réponses exactes et complètes à toutes les questions de la présente demande |
|----|----|

D - J   M   Y - A

_____     _____
Signature of applicant - Signature du requérant            Date

IMM 1295 (06-2002) B

## 6.5       OVERSEAS WORKERS

### 6.5.1  CONSULAR OFFICE IN CANADA

➢ As a new caregiver in Canada, it is important that you look through the phone book for the nearest consular office of your country of origin.  Remember that for the next two years, you are only considered a visitor to Canada with an employment status. There are many ethnic organizations that you also should be in contact with for your acculturation and settlement.

➢ SICES CANADA ALUMNI ASSOCIATION is responsible for your welfare during your first 24 months of employment. For example, finding a new employer, moving from province to province or taking care of you while unemployed. Remember that you cannot work for a new prospective employer unless your change of employer status is confirmed. SICES Alumni has respite homes for caregivers. If you are not a SICES graduate, SICES Canada will assist you in your acculturation as part of its commitment to assist newcomers to Canada.

➢ Upon arriving in Canada you are requested to register at SICES Canada through telephone.

Toll Free: All parts of Canada  - 1-800-577-4267
Within Edmonton, Alberta - (780) 474-4900
Or email your registration to sicesca@telus.net

➢ You are to provide the following information:
- Name
- Current Address
- Telephone Number
- Date of Arrival

This information is for SICES Alumni Association's use because during the first two years, it is important that SICES members have a resource association to turn to.

### 6.5.2  APPLYING FOR A S.I.N.

➢ The S.I.N. (Social Insurance Number) is a 9 digit identification number used by Government Programs in Canada. You cannot work in Canada or receive government benefits without a S.I.N.

### Process of Getting S.I.N.

1. You are required to fill out a S.I.N. application form which is available at any local Human Resource Development Center (HDRC) or can be downloaded from the HRDC web page "http://www.hrdc-drhc.gc.ca".

2. A primary document and secondary document is required to be submitted along with the application form. The primary document proves your identity and status in Canada.

   *Examples of primary documents*:
   - Birth certificates
   - Permit to Come into or Remain in Canada/Temporary Resident Permit
   - Student Authorization/Study Permit
   - Visitor Record, Extension of Permit/Extension to Temporary Resident Permit
   - Determination of Eligibility/Consideration of Eligibility
   - Consideration of Eligibility and CIC letter.

3. A secondary document is required only if the name on your primary document is different from the name you legally use.

   Examples of valid secondary documents
   - Marriage Certificates
   - Divorce Decrees
   - Legal Change of Name Documents
   - Declaration of Assumed Name/Statutory Declarations
   - Adoption Papers
   - Request to Amend Immigration Record of Landing.

4. Original copies of both primary and secondary documents must be submitted.

It is advisable to apply for your SIN in person rather than sending your application by mail. The accidental loss of your identification papers by mail may be avoided. For more information of applying for a S.I.N. go to "http://www.hrdc-drhc.gc.ca".

In Edmonton, you can access SICES hotline (780) 474-4900 to walk you through the various forms to be filled in like S.I.N. and Alberta Health Care.

### 6.5.3  COORDINATION WITH THE CIC

(Source: Citizenship and Immigration Canada)

### *THE LIVE IN CAREGIVER PROGRAM*
> ➢ The Live In Caregiver Program is an opportunity for qualified caregivers to work in Canada in situations where there is a lack of Canadians to fill positions. Live-in caregivers are qualified individuals that provide care for the elderly, children, and people with disabilities. Live-in caregivers are to work in private homes and must live with their employer.

### *ELIGIBILITY FOR THE LIVE IN CAREGIVER PROGRAM*
> ➢ Completed course work that is equivalent to a Canadian secondary school diploma.
> ➢ Completed a 6 month full-time training course in a classroom setting or worked 12 months in a full time job that relates to the caregiving job that is being sought through the live-in caregiver program.
> ➢ Write and speak fluent English or French.
> ➢ Must have a written contract with a future employer.

Caregivers under the live-in caregiver program can only work for the employer stated on their working permit. The working permit is only valid for one year and must be renewed with a written letter from the employer stating continued employment for the following year.

In the case of changing employers, a new work permit must be obtained that states the name of the new employer. A written contract with the new employer is required to obtain a new permit.

Permanent resident status can be obtained after an equivalent of two years as a live-in caregiver. This must be completed within three years after first arriving in Canada and can span multiple employers but must have worked for one employer at a time.

# HOW TO'S

*Julie V. Kallal*

# Individual Task Practice (ITP)How to Take Vital Signs

## A. TEMPERATURE
### 1. Equipment
- oral or rectal thermometer (normal rdg: oral (37°C) rectum (37.5)
- cotton balls
- soap

### 2. Oral
- wash hands
- wipe the thermometer by the end opposite the mercury bulb
- wipe the thermometer with a cotton ball dipped in water to remove any antiseptic solution
- shake the thermometer down so that the mercury register 35 degrees Celsius
- place the bulb between the lips and under the tongue
- make sure the mouth is closed
- allow about three minutes for thermometer to register oral temperature change.
- to take accurate reading, leave the thermometer in the mouth for 8 to 10 minutes
- to read the temperature, slowly roll it backwards and forwards until the end of the mercury column can be seen clearly
- wash hands and record the temperature

### 3. Rectal
- wash hands
- ask the person to lie on his side with his bottom leg straight
- ask the person to flex his upper leg over the bottom leg
- shake the thermometer down 35°C and gently insert into the rectum about 2.5 cm deep
- keep the thermometer in place between 3 to 5 minutes
- remove the thermometer gently, read the person's temperature
- disinfect the thermometer and wash hands
- record the person's temperature

## B. PULSE
- the person should be at rest for at least 20 minutes
- place 2 to 3 fingers on the inside of the older person's wrist just below the back of his thumb
- do not use a thumb in taking the pulse as it has a pulse of its own
- press lightly on the artery with 2 fingers being careful not to stop blood flow
- using the second hand of a watch, count the beats in 60 seconds duration

## C. RESPIRATION
- count the number of respiration cycles (breathe in, breathe out, pause) over 60 second period and record

# ITP 2 <u>How to Assist in Giving Medication</u>

In order to avoid errors in administering medications and possible adverse drug reaction, hospitalization and even death, the following FIVE RIGHTS OF GIVING MEDICATION must be observed at all times when administering any kind of medication:

    1.  right medication
    2.  right person
    3.  right amount
    4.  right time
    5.  right method

An easier way to remember the five rights is by thinking **"MPATM" (medication, person, amount, time, method)**. *Think of the MM candy and pat on your belly.*

## 1. Right Medication

Check medication carefully, then check the label of the container making sure that you have the right medication.

## 2. Right Person

Do not administer any prescribed medication to anyone other than the person for whom it was prescribed, no matter how similar the illness may seem- in other words give the right medication to the right person only.

## 3. Right Amount

Don't play doctor. Always count or measure the prescribed dosage precisely and accurately – no more, no less. Give only the amount of right medication to the right person.

## 4. Right Time

It is important to give the right amount of the right medication to the right person at the right time. Read label, the label indicates the time.

## 5. Right Method

The right method on the label will specify whether the medication is to be taken or applied to the skin or given in drops using a medicine dropper.

# ITP 3 <u>How to Administer Topical Medications</u>

The most common topical medications are nose drops or sprays, ear drops, eye drops and skin applications.

## *NOSE DROPS*
1. Wash hands.
2. Read the label to ensure the right medication.
3. Ask the person to lie flat on his bed.
4. Read the label again before filling the dropper with the right dosage.
5. Drop the nose drops into the nose making sure that the dropper does not touch the nostril of the person.
6. Repeat steps 4 and 5 if medication is required into the other nostril.
7. Ask the person to remain flat for at least one minute to retain the drops in the nose.
8. Wash hands and record time, medicine and dosage.

## *NASAL SPRAYS*
Use the nose drops procedure except that the person should be sitting and keeping his head upright while the medication is being sprayed into each nostril.

> **Caution:** Avoid using nasal spray after three days because of the contamination of the spray nozzle.

## *ORAL MEDICATIONS*
Oral medications may take the form of tablets, capsules or liquid. They are usually best taken by the person in a sitting position. A sip of water before administering the medication may be helpful.

### *Tablet or Capsule Form*
1. Wash your hands.
2. Read the label for the right medication.
3. Just before putting the capsule or tablet in a medicine cup, read the label again.
4. Giving the cup with medicine in, the person with one hand, hold the container in the other and read the label to the person.
5. Give medication with large glass of water or whatever is indicated by the doctor on the label.
6. Wash your hands and record the time, the medicine and the amount given.

### Liquid Form

1.  Wash hands.
2.  Read the label for the right medication.
3.  Mix the contents of the bottle by gently turning the container from the top to bottom unless instructed to shake the container vigorously. Roll the container back and forth between your hands.
4.  Read the label again before measuring the exact dosage.
5.  Pour the medicine into the medicine cup at eye level.
6.  Check the label once more before giving the medication to the right person.
7.  Ensure that the person swallows all the medicine.
8.  Wash hands and record medicine, time and dosage.

# ITP 4 <u>How to Administer Rectal Medications</u>

Suppositories and enemas are two medications that are administered rectally.

## *RECTAL SUPPOSITORY*

1.  Wash hands.
2.  Follow the direction on the package carefully.
3.  To administer, have the person lie down on his side with the upper knee flexed over the lower leg.
4.  Put on disposable gloves, remove the wrapper from the suppository and discard wrapper.
5.  Insert the suppository into the rectum about 2.5 cm with the pointed end first.
6.  The effect of the suppository will become noticeable in about 20 minutes.
7.  Wash hands and record time, medicine and results.

## *ENEMA*

1.  Wash hands.
2.  Keep the enema solution at room temperature.
3.  Encourage the person to use bathroom before administering enema.
4.  Have the person lie down on his left side with the upper knee flexed over the lower leg.
5.  Place a protective sheet (plastic sheet) under the buttock of the person.
6.  Lubricate the nozzle, gently insert into the rectum (approximately 5-8 cms).
7.  Gently release all of the enema solution into the rectum.
8.  Wash hands and record time, drug and results.

## ITP 5 <u>How to Reduce Fever</u>

There are three ways in which to reduce fever:

1. Drink plenty of fluids.
2. Have the person take a tepid bath or shower.
3. Give the person a tepid sponge bath.

However, the following precautions must be observed before administering any of the above:

1. Avoid sponging with ice cold or hot water.
2. When dealing with an older person, always check with a health professional giving plenty of fluids especially in cases where the elderly is taking water or heart pills or on a salt restricted diet.
3. Always record the temperature, pulse and respirations before and after administering a tepid sponge bath.
4. If the person starts to shiver, cover him and wait until the shivering stops (shivering occurs because the body temperature is falling too rapidly and the body is losing too much heat quickly. It is the body's defense mechanism against heat loss).
5. Always consult a doctor if fever persists or if the body temperature has not dropped within an hour.

# ITP 6 <u>How to Give A Bath</u>

## *TEPID SPONGE BATH*

1. Wash hands.
2. Record temperature, pulse and respirations.
3. Bathe the front and back of body using long even strokes.
4. Use a towel to cover the body to prevent shivering.
5. Place tepid water soaked towel on areas where the blood vessels are close to the surface (under the arms, back of neck, the wrists and in the groin).
6. Change towels frequently.
7. Dry the person thoroughly.
8. Replace wet bedding as required.
9. Wash the person's hands.
10. Record the person's temperature, pulse and respirations after 20 minutes.
11. If tub bath is preferred instead, the procedure is the same except that soap is not used.
12. The entire bath should not last more than twenty minutes.

# ITP 7 <u>How to Assist in Dressing Up</u>

1.  Encourage the person to do much of the dressing procedure as possible.
2.  Use only loose fitting garments and clothing that are easy to put or take off.
3.  Place clothing within reach of the person.
4.  If person is sitting up, slip the garment over the head first.
5.  If the arms are weak, the clothing should be put into the sleeves first.
6.  Encourage the person to button up, zip up or fasten hooks by himself/herself.
7.  If the person is lying down, slip the arms into the clothing first and ease the neck opening over the head.
8.  If one arm is immobilized, dress that arm first by slipping a hand through the sleeve of the garment and grasping the weak hand.
9.  When dressing the lower part of the body, pull the pants or trousers over the feet and up the legs, then ease the clothing over the hips while the person attempts to lift his body off the bed.
10. If the person is unable to lift himself then assist him roll over one side. Pull the pants or trousers farthest away from the bed over his hip. Roll him to the other side and repeat procedure.

## ITP 8 <u>How to Make a Bed</u>

### WHEN BED IS OCCUPIED

1. Wash hands.
2. Position a chair at the foot of the bed.
3. Ask the person to lie flat if possible.
4. Remove the bedspread, blankets and extra pillow. Leave only the top sheet as cover for the person.
5. Position the person on one side and keep him covered with the top sheet.
6. Use a chair to prevent the person from rolling off the bed.
7. Move to the other side of the bed. Roll soiled bottom sheet toward the centre of the bed.
8. Lay a clean sheet, folded lengthwise on the bed with the folded side toward the centre of the bed.
9. Lay the draw sheet, folded in half, on the bed with the folded side toward the centre of the bed.
10. Tuck the sheet under the head of the mattress and make a mitred corner.
11. Starting from the head to the foot of the bed, tuck the side of the sheet under the mattress.
12. Make another mitred corner at the foot of the bed.
13. Tuck in the draw sheet.
14. Reposition the person to the other side of the bed. Ensure the person does not fall off. Move the chair to the other side of the bed.
15. Remove soiled bottom sheet, unfold the sheets and tuck them in.
16. Assist the person to a comfortable position and replace cover sheet.
17. Replace the blankets and bedspread cover sheet.
18. Change pillow cases.
19. Remove soiled linens to the laundry room.
20. Wash hands.

# ITP 9 <u>How to Lift Heavy Objects Off the Floor</u>

Lifting happens all the time and if you are not careful, it may lead to unnecessary pain and sometimes disability.

1. Bend the knees
2. Grasp the object with both hands.
3. Use the muscles from your thighs to get you in the position.
4. Try balancing the object and before lifting gauge your strength against it.
5. Never lift objects that are too heavy. Wait to get some help.
6. Always have your feet flat on the floor. Tip toeing is not a good practice.

## ITP 10      How to Transfer a Person to a Chair or Wheelchair

In executing this transfer procedure, ensure that you use slow and steady movements allowing the person time and energy to adjust and prepare himself to help you along the way. Be sure to control each step by pausing between each step.

1. Ask the person to place his legs at the edge of the bed.
2. Face the person, put one foot in front of the other and place your elbow closest to the bed on the bed.
3. Bend both knees and grasp the person above his elbow.
4. Ask the person to grasp your arms.
5. Using your arm lever and rocking back on your heels, instructing the person to pull up, assist him in a sitting position.
6. Assist him to lower his legs and put on foot wear.
7. Place a chair sideways next to the bed.
8. Assist him to slide forward to the edge of the bed.
9. Stand in front of the person, hold onto hid waist while he holds onto your shoulders.
10. Bend at the knees, place your knee farthest away from the chair against his corresponding knee.
11. Pivot the person towards the chair and lower him onto the chair or wheelchair.

# ITP 11    How to Position a Person in Bed (4 Positions)

### *TO MOVE UP IN BED*
1. Remove pillows and ask the person to lie flat.
2. Bend knees and feet flat on bed.
3. Stand directly behind the head of the person's bed.
4. Ask the person to fold his arms across his chest.
5. Reach under the armpits and grasp the wrists.
6. Bend at your knees and use your knees as levers against the bed. MAKE SURE TO USE PROPER BODY MECHANISM WHILE ASSISTING.
7. Tell the person that as pull, he must down on the bed with both feet. Then in one movement, pull him up.
8. Replace the pillows.
   Note: Step 7 can be used to move a person in a chair or up in that chair or wheelchair.

### *TO MOVE A PERSON TO A BACK-LYING POSITION IN BED*
1. When a person gets tired of being in a side-lying position, he can be positioned onto his back.
2. Stand at the side of the bed not facing the person.
3. Remove any pillows.
4. Place one of your feet infront of the other and bend your knees.
5. Place one hand on the person's upper shoulder and one hand on the upper hip.
6. Roll the person onto his back by shifting your weight from the front to the back foot.
7. Line up the person's head, shoulders and hips.
8. Replace pillows.

### *TO MOVE A PERSON TO THE SIDE-LYING POSITION IN BED*
1. Stand opposite the person's waist on the side of the bed to which the person wishes to be turned.
2. Ask the person to place his arm farthest away from you cross his chest.
3. Ask the person to bend his leg farthest away from you and keep foot flat on the bed.
4. Place one of your feet in front of the other.
5. Place one hand on the shoulder farthest from you and other hand on the hip farthest from you.
6. Bend at the knees and roll the person towards you while shifting your weight from the front to the back foot.
7. Assist the person to achieve the most comfortable position by placing the pillows, adjusting clothing, bending knees, straightening feet, etc.

## *THE SITTING POSITION IN BED*

1. In a sitting position, place the person at about 45 degree angle with his back supported by pillow or backrest.
2. Try to create a hollow between the shoulders and the lower back while arranging the pillows to enable the person to breathe more easily.

# ITP 12    How to Transfer a Person From a Fall/Bathtub

In some cases, senior or disabled person may become weak during a transfer procedure. Therefore, the following steps are recommended:

## *FROM A FALL*

1. If the person is suddenly becomes weak while in a transfer, gradually lower him to the floor while bending at the knees.
2. Check if the person is hurt or unconscious.
3. If hurt or unconscious, activate medical aid.
4. Apply first aid.
5. Prevent shock and keep him warm.
6. If unhurt, place a chair in front of the person to assist and support him.
7. Make sure the chair is sturdy and immobilized.
8. Stand behind the person and bend at the knees.
9. Gradually help the person to a standing position by placing one arm under the person's arm and the other arm around his waist.
10. Turn him around.
11. Lower him to the chair.

## *IN OR OUT OF THE BATHTUB*

1. Place a non-skid mat in the bottom of the tub.
2. Test the temperature of the water.
3. Encourage the person to use grab bars.
4. Discourage the use of shower curtain or soap dish handle as a lever in getting in or out of the tub.
5. If the person prefers to sit during his bath or shower, a small tool may be used, however, always asses the balance and muscle strength of the person to determine the need for such tools.
6. Assist the person to face towards the shower head or tap.
7. Stand beside the person and support his side farthest away from the tub.
8. Bend at the knees.
9. While supporting the person, tell him to place one leg in the tub.
10. Encourage him to use the grab bar for balance as he places the other leg in the tub.
11. Provide support as the person sits on the stool.
12. Place a towel under the person's arms while assisting him to lower himself into the tub.
13. When finished, drain the water out of the tub.
14. If the person is sitting, wrap the person's upper body in the bath towel.
15. Encourage the person to use grab bar during the lifting procedure.

16. Bend at the knees and provide support as the person transfer to a standing position and out of the tub.
17. If lying down, run a towel under the person's arms and assist him to a standing position and out of the tub.

# ITP 13    How to Give a Back Rub

Every kind of massage is geared to relieving tension, relaxing muscles and increasing the oxygen-carrying capacity of the blood. Swedish massage involved kneading and tapping individual muscles to stimulate nerves. An oriental massage, known as *Shiatsu*, works on the principle of energy balance. Finger pressures, some light, some heavy, are thought to break down the blockage of energy. A back rub helps a bedridden to relieve the building pressures on his back and relaxes the individual.

Check the room temperature and avoid possible drafts and wash hands before and after each back rub.

1. Use a body cream or Vaseline oil to prevent too much friction.
2. Divide the back mentally into four sections.
3. Work on section at a time, kneading the muscles between your hands, alternate using fingers and palms of your hands. You may also use the edges of your hands to stimulate a chopping motion.
4. Go u p and down the spine with your forefinger and middle finger and use circular motion on each vertebrate.
5. Finally, wash your hands.

## ITP 14     How to Shampoo a Bedridden Person

You will need:
* a garbage bag with a hole for the head     * a tub or bucket
* a plastic sheet for the bed     * wash cloth
* some large towels     * shampoo

### PROCEDURE:

1. Set the temperature of the room at 24 degrees Celsius.
2. Protect the bed with a plastic sheet.
3. Protect the body of the person with plastic bag.
4. Assist the person into position by placing pillows under the shoulders and the person's head hanging at the edge of the bed.
5. Protect the person's eye with a wash cloth.
6. Place a tub or bucket under the person's head.
7. Pour some water over the hair, rub some shampoo in and massage the scalp and hair.
8. Rinse the hair several times.
9. Dry hair thoroughly by towel drying or with the use of a hair dryer.
10. Cleans up and wash hands.

# ITP 15    How to Assist During Exercise

## *DEEP BREATHING EXERCISE*

1. Wash hands.
2. Assist person into a sitting position or by supporting upper body with pillows.
3. Do not stand directly in front of the person during the breathing exercises to avoid exposure to droplets carrying germs that may be exhaled or coughed up by the person.
4. Have the person place his/her hands on either side of the rib cage so that expansion and contraction can be left.
5. Ask the person to breathe in through his nose and hold hi breath for 3 seconds.
6. Encourage the person to use the muscles of the chest to breathe in.
7. After 3 seconds ask the person to breathe out through his mouth only.
8. Repeat the exercise 10 times and at least once a day.
9. Encourage the person to cough up any mucus during breathing out part of the exercise. Always have some tissues available and a small plastic film to wrap the soiled tissues before placing them in the garbage bag.
10. Always wash hands at the end (you and the person).

## *EXERCISING THE LEGS AND FEET*

1. Rotate the ankles ten times.
2. Flex and extend the toes of the feet.
3. Bend both knees slightly, then extend the legs as far as they can go. Push feet against some firm objects – wall, foot board.
4. Repeat ten times.
5. Bend both knees and maintain a semi-sitting position for 5 seconds. Repeat 5 times.
6. Do the above exercises once a day.

## ITP 16    How to Prepare or Apply Cold or Hot Applications

Heat or cold compress may be applied to the skin for therapeutic reasons. Dry heat may be applied to the skin in the form of an electric pad, electric blanket or hot water bottle. Moist heat may be applied to the skin in the form of a hot bath, hot shower, moist compresses, foot soak, sitz bath or tepid sponge bath. Dry cold may be applied to the skin in the form of ice pack or ice bag. Moist cold may be applied to the skin in the form of compresses made out of folded towels.

### *HEAT APPLICATION*
**Hot Water Bottle:**   Test the hot water bottle for leaks by filling it with water, screwing the top on and tipping it upside down.

1.   Add 2 parts of hot to 1 part of cold water making sure the temperature is tolerate to the hand.
2.   Place the hot water bottle in a sink and pour the water up to the 2/3 full mark.
3.   Press down on the sides of the bottle to make the water rise to the top, expelling air inside the bottle.
4.   Screw the top of the hot water bottle and test for leaks again.
5.   Wrap the hot water bottle in a towel and place on the affected area of the skin.
6.   Check the skin frequently for signs of burning or pain or discomfort.
7.   Remove the hot water bottle after the prescribed time and record the effect of the application.

**Heating Pad:**       Ensure that the heating pad is in proper working condition.

1.   Pre-heat the heating pad to the desired control. If there is a doctor's order then pre-set control to the prescribed order.
2.   Apply the heating pad to the affected area and monitor the skin frequently for pain, discomfort or burns.
3.   Remove the heating pad after the prescribed time and record effects of applications.

**Warm and Moist Compress:**    If the doctor orders, warm and moist compresses may be applied to affected area of the skin when the skin is not broken.

1.   Pour heated water into a bucket or basin where a folded towel or face cloth are  placed previously.
2.   Lift one compress on the affected area and cover with a towel.
3.   Apply one compress on the affected area and cover with a towel.
4.   Monitor skin for any sign of discomfort or burning and repeat applications

of warm and moist compresses as required.

5. Wash hands and record effects of application.

**Moist Heat:** Moist heat may be administered in the form of sitz bath, foot soak, sponge bath or showers. In the case of sitz bath, a doctor should be consulted.

## *COLD APPLICATION*

**Ice Pack:** Ice pack or ice therapy is also known as CRYOTHERAPY. The most important rule to remember when doing any kind of activity is to stop immediately as soon as you experience any kind of pain. Pain is not pressure. Pain is anything that you feel that is not normal.

1. Use a bag of frozen corn, peas or mixed vegetables. Ice cubes in a bag also work but are not as effective as the frozen vegetable bag. Make sure to label the frozen gab so as not to mistake it fro food.
2. Take frozen bag and wrap it in a damp towel or terry cloth.
3. Apply it on the affected area for a maximum of 20 minutes. Allow the area to warm up on its own.
4. Re-apply after an hour and continue to use every other hour as needed to control pain.
5. If the person is suffering from a low back pain, do not lay him on the ice pack. Chilling works better, so encourage the person to walk around with the bag in place. If the person prefers to sit, then sit in a straight backed chair, not in a recliner or soft chair.

**Cold Moist Compress:** A doctor may sometimes prescribed cold moist compresses

1. Place a folded face towel in a bowl of ice and water.
2. Place a dry towel over the affected area.
3. Wring out a compress to remove excess water.
4. Apply to the affected area.
5. Continue the above procedure until the prescribed time.
6. Monitor the underlying skin for signs of blueness and/or numbness. Discontinue therapy if any of these signs occur.
7. Clean up area, wash hands and record effects of application.
   Report numbness or blueness immediately to the health professional.

## ITP 17    How to Feed a Bedridden Person

Bedridden persons who are partially dependent should encourage to help themselves during the feeding procedure. Give the person a chance to freshen up – comb hair, wash hands, rinse mouth, use bed pan or washroom, etc.

1. If able to sit up, provide pillows or backrest for support. If not, place him in the side-lying position (see ITP 12).
2. Wash hands (yours and his)
3. Place a bib or towel across his chest to protect his clothing.
4. Test hot food by scooping a small amount in a spoon especially fluid. Do not use straws for hot soup or fluid.
5. Use utensils normally used for the food being eaten.
6. Advise the person what is on the tray and encourage him to feed himself as much as possible.
7. Offer fluid often. Either use a feeder cup, a normal glass or straws (cold fluid) if he is not prone to gas accumulation.
8. Take time during the feeding procedure. Serve bite size portions and let him decide when the next bite is to be served.
9. Try to avoid spillage. Wipe mouth and chin when necessary. Be very careful when doing any wiping as it may be upsetting to the person.
10. Try to have a pleasant topic for conversation during the feeding procedure.
11. Avoid over feeding and clean up area after feeding.
12. Perform mouth care, wash face, offer bedpan.
13. Wash hands (yours and the person requiring care).

## *ABOUT THE AUTHOR*

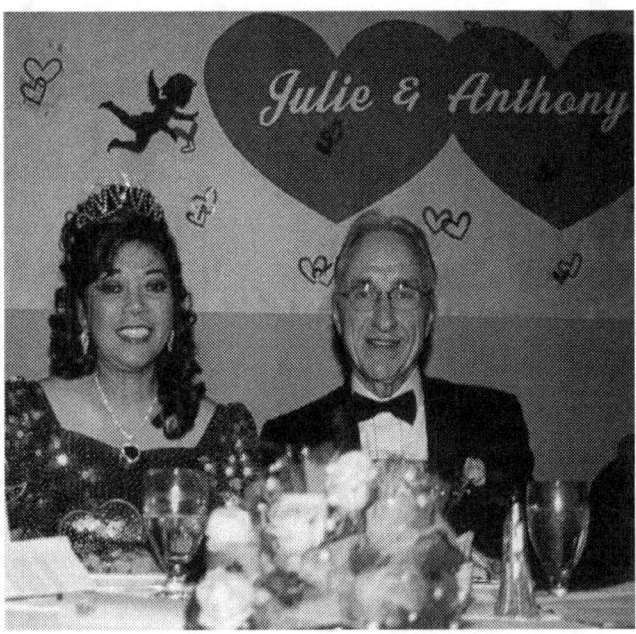

**Julie with husband Anthony**

## Julieta Valeriano Kallal

Just so you know who I am. In 1967, I came to Canada and
Uprooted myself from my native county, the most beautiful,
Lovely and exotic Philippines. FYI, I am the eldest girl
In the family of eight. My husband and I have now been
Enjoying life, by involving ourselves in many ways, in
The real pleasures of living as society's antique treasures.
As a member of life-long learning, I really have a lot to say.

Vigorously accepting many challenges in this chaotic life,
Accepting many issues involving various critical human
Life problems, I, for one, have been blessed with an
Excellent competency to assist individuals in many
Rural and urban settings worldwide. There are topics &
Issues such as care giving skills, health, safety, English
As a Second Language training, high school courses
Nurturing and cultural resources that need to be
Overcome and I'm proud to be part of the solutions.

Keen on contributing to individuals' social, physical
Academic, creative, cultural, economic and emotional
Lives and enhancement, I have devoted my day to day
Living in seriously designing, developing, implementing
And evaluating programs and activities that will surely
Lend themselves to a worthy donation to life itself!

www.ingramcontent.com/pod-product-compliance
Lightning Source LLC
Chambersburg PA
CBHW081107170526
45165CB00008B/2360